Comprehensive Atlas of Transplantation

Comprehensive Atlas of Transplantation

Editors

■ Paul C. Kuo

Professor of Surgery
Department of Surgery
Duke University Medical Center
Durham, North Carolina

■ R. Duane Davis

Associate Professor of Surgery
Department of Surgery
Duke University Medical Center
Durham, North Carolina

Associate Editors

■ Donald C. Dafoe, MD

Samuel D. Gross Professor and Chairman
Department of Surgery
Thomas Jefferson University Hospital
Philadelphia, Pennsylvania

■ R. Randal Bollinger

Professor of Surgery
Department of Surgery
Duke University Medical Center
Durham, North Carolina

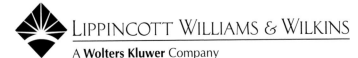

LIPPINCOTT WILLIAMS & WILKINS
A **Wolters Kluwer** Company

Philadelphia • Baltimore • New York • London
Buenos Aires • Hong Kong • Sydney • Tokyo

Acquisitions Editor: Craig Percy
Developmental Editor: Maureen Iannuzzi
Supervising Editor: Melanie Bennitt
Production Editor: Helen Powers
Manufacturing Manager: Benjamin Rivera
Cover Designer: Karen Quigley
Compositor: Maryland Composition
Printer: Kingsport

© 2005 by **LIPPINCOTT WILLIAMS & WILKINS**
530 Walnut Street
Philadelphia, PA 19106 USA
LWW.com

Printed in the USA

Library of Congress Cataloging-in-Publication Data

Comprehensive atlas of transplantation / editors, Paul C. Kuo, R. Duane Davis; associate editors, Donald C. Dafoe, R. Randall Bollinger.
    p. ; cm.
  Includes bibliographical references and index.
  ISBN 0-7817-4497-0
  1. Transplantation of organs, tissues, etc.—Atlases. I. Kuo, Paul C. II. Davis, R. Duane.
  [DNLM: 1. Transplantation—Atlases. WO 517 C7376 2005]
  RD120.7.C644 2005
  617.9′5—dc22

2004013936

Care has been taken to confirm the accuracy of the information presented and to describe generally accepted practices. However, the authors, editors, and publisher are not responsible for errors or omissions or for any consequences from application of the information in this book and make no warranty, expressed or implied, with respect to the currency, completeness, or accuracy of the contents of the publication. Application of this information in a particular situation remains the professional responsibility of the practitioner.

    The authors, editors, and publisher have exerted every effort to ensure that drug selection and dosage set forth in this text are in accordance with current recommendations and practice at the time of publication. However, in view of ongoing research, changes in government regulations, and the constant flow of information relating to drug therapy and drug reactions, the reader is urged to check the package insert for each drug for any change in indications and dosage and for added warnings and precautions. This is particularly important when the recommended agent is a new or infrequently employed drug.

    Some drugs and medical devices presented in this publication have Food and Drug Administration (FDA) clearance for limited use in restricted research settings. It is the responsibility of the health care provider to ascertain the FDA status of each drug or device planned for use in their clinical practice.

10 9 8 7 6 5 4 3 2 1

*To the many residents in surgery and fellows in transplantation
who have contributed to the knowledge that we share in this atlas.*

Contents

Contributing Authors

R. Randal Bollinger, MD, PhD
Department of Surgery,
Duke University Medical Center,
Durham, North Carolina

William C. Chapman, MD
Department of Surgery,
Washington University School of
Medicine,
St. Louis, Missouri

Bradley H. Collins, MD
Department of Surgery,
Duke University Medical Center,
Durham, North Carolina

Donald C. Dafoe, MD
Department of Surgery,
Thomas Jefferson University Hospital,
Philadelphia, Pennsylvania

R. Duane Davis, MD
Department of Surgery,
Duke University Medical Center,
Durham, North Carolina

Niraj M. Desai, MD
Department of Surgery,
Washington University School of
Medicine,
St. Louis, Missouri

Matthew G. Hartwig, MD
Department of Surgery,
Duke University Medical Center,
Durham, North Carolina

Martin Jendrisak, MD
Department of Surgery,
Washington University School of
Medicine,
St. Louis, Missouri

Reena C. Jha, MD
Department of Radiology,
Georgetown University Hospital,
Washington, DC

Lynt B. Johnson, MD
Department of Surgery,
Georgetown University Hospital,
Transplant Institute,
Washington, DC

Paul C. Kuo, MD, MBA
Department of Surgery,
Duke University Medical Center,
Durham, North Carolina

Shu S. Lin, MD, PhD
Department of Surgery,
Duke University Medical Center,
Durham, North Carolina

Jeffrey A. Lowell, MD
Department of Surgery,
Washington University School of
Medicine,
St. Louis, Missouri

Amy D. Lu, MD
Department of Surgery,
Georgetown University Hospital,
Transplant Institute,
Washington, DC

Carlos E. Marroquin, MD
Department of Surgery,
Duke University Medical Center,
Durham, North Carolina

Carmelo A. Milano, MD
Department of Surgery,
Duke University Medical Cener,
Durham, North Carolina

Jason A. Petrofski, MD
Department of Surgery,
Duke University Medical Center,
Durham, North Carolina

James J. Pomposelli, MD, PhD
Department of Surgery,
Lahey Clinic Medical Center,
Burlington, Massachusetts

Elizabeth A. Pomfret, MD, PhD
Department of Surgery,
Lahey Clinic Medical Center,
Burlington, Massachusetts

Lloyd E. Ratner, MD
Department of Surgery,
Thomas Jefferson University Hospital,
Philadelphia, Pennsylvania

John E. Scarborough, MD
Department of Surgery,
Duke University Medical Center
Durham, North Carolina

Rebecca A. Schroeder, MD
Department of Anesthesiology,
Duke University Medical Center,
Durham, North Carolina

Surendra Shenoy, MD, PhD
Department of Surgery,
Washington University School of
Medicine,
St. Louis, Missouri

Ross W. Shepherd, MD
Department of Surgery,
Washington University School of
Medicine,
St. Louis, Missouri

Sinan A. Simsir, MD
Department of Surgery,
Duke University Medical Center,
Durham, North Carolina

Steven S.L. Tsui, MA, MD, FRCS
Consultant Cardiothoracic Surgeon,
Papworth Hospital,
Cambridge, United Kingdom

J. Elizabeth Tuttle-Newhall, MD
Department of Surgery,
Duke University Medical Center,
Durham, North Carolina

Foreword

Drs. Kuo and Davis have assembled a talented team of authors and co-authors to produce a new atlas of transplant surgery, *Comprehensive Atlas of Transplantation*. Not only does their book cover the full spectrum of surgical techniques used to transplant solid organs, but it also concisely summarizes the fundamental principles of organ preservation and multi-organ procurement. In separate chapters, leaders in the field describe and discuss the state-of-the art for heart, lung, liver, kidney, and pancreas transplantation. Given the importance of living donation for patients with end-organ failure and the burgeoning interest in this type of transplantation, the sections of their atlas that address operative strategies for harvesting liver and kidney from living donors are particularly valuable. In all sections, their overall approach is unique because of the use of digital photography for imaging that greatly enhances and enriches the visual displays of operative technique. I have no doubt that this text will be a valuable resource for resident physicians, fellows, and established surgeons as well as for our colleagues-in-training in the allied health professions. As such, I am delighted and honored to introduce you to their master work.

Danny O. Jacobs, MD, MPH
Chairman, Department of Surgery
Duke University Medical Center
Durham, North Carolina

Preface

The *Comprehensive Atlas of Transplantation* is intended to provide a step-by-step pictorial guide to performing state-of-the-art transplant procedures. This atlas is unique in that it addresses transplant procedures in thoracic and abdominal compartments, includes living-donor procedures for both liver and kidney, and utilizes digital photography to convey pictorial representations. In addition, a section addressing organ procurement and management of the multi-organ cadaver donor is included. It is our intent that students, residents, and practitioners in transplant surgery will find this book of great use. We have firmly committed to providing a thorough perspective on state-of-the-art transplant procedures. Howeve, we recognize that many successful variations exist for surgical transplant techniques. By no means are the procedures in this atlas meant to represent the sole approach for performing these procedures. We sincerely hope that this work will be of assistance in the training of future transplant surgeons and physicians.

It is a privilege to present this work to the surgical community. We wish to thank Maureen Iannuzzi, Brian Brown, and Lippincott Williams & Wilkins for their tireless efforts in bringing this work to fruition.

Paul C. Kuo, MD
R. Duane Davis, MD

Section I

Multi-Organ Procurement

Chapter 1

Management Considerations in the Multi-Organ Donor

■ **Rebecca A. Schroeder, M.D.**

Department of Anesthesiology, Duke University
Medical Center, Durham, NC

At the time of declaration of brain death, management goals for the patient are changed dramatically from preserving life and neurologic function to preserving and optimizing the function of specific organs at the expense of other systems. On a general level, basic critical care principles remain the same, but a different balance must be struck that takes into account which organs are being considered for procurement and transplantation.

Optimizing cardiovascular system function can be a challenging task, frequently made more complicated if the thoracic organs are being considered for transplantation. Stresses of enormous proportion accompany the evolution of brain death itself, not to mention the negative consequences that treatment of severe neurologic injury may involve. Significant volume depletion from mannitol and other diuretic therapies aimed at minimizing intracranial pressure and the consequences of the catecholamine surge and subsequent deficit often leave the potential donor hypotensive and inotrope-dependent. Myocardial dysfunction results from excessive inotrope use, brain death physiology, or severe hypovolemia. Fluid resuscitation guided by central venous monitoring or even pulmonary artery catheter placement is mandatory, with the goal of reducing the dependence of the patient on inotropes for maintenance of systolic arterial blood pressure greater than 90 to 100 mm Hg. Colloids or crystalloids may be used for volume repletion to achieve a central venous pressure of 9 to 12 mm Hg. Nonglucose-containing solutions should be used to avoid hyperglycemia and resulting osmotic diuresis. A pulmonary artery catheter may be indicated to evaluate thoracic organs for donation or due to coexisting medical conditions in the donor such as valvular disease, cardiomyopathy, severe lung disease, or persistent hypotension.

Hypotension resistant to fluid repletion is common among organ donors and is most frequently treated with peripheral vasoconstrictors. Dopamine has been the pressor of choice, presumably due to its mesenteric vasodilating capabilities, although this has not been documented in humans. The use of inotropes is discouraged by many centers due to concerns of catecholamine-induced cardiomyopathy in the donor, as well as catecholamine depletion of the myocardium due to endogenous catecholamine release with attenuation of responses to subsequent catecholamine administration. In addition, high doses of vasopressor agents decrease blood flow to vital organs, possibly resulting in ischemic injury to those very organs intended for transplant. In general, low doses of dopamine (less than 7.5 μg/kg/min) are considered acceptable. Further vasopressor therapy must be guided by invasive monitoring assistance. The addition of arginine vasopressin may also be considered at this point. Unrestrained use of fluid to maintain acceptable organ perfusion, however, must be balanced against the risk of inducing volume overload and pulmonary edema. This would disqualify the lungs for potential donation, in addition to potentially impairing gas exchange and causing arterial hypoxemia and end-organ ischemia.

Additional cardiovascular issues requiring attention include arrhythmias and sudden cardiac arrest. In a review of brain-dead patients maintained on ventilators, 62% suffered cardiac arrest within 24 hours, while 87% did so within 72 hours. Atropine in the brain-dead patient is ineffective, and direct beta-agonists such as isoproterenol or epinephrine are necessary. In addition, other injuries such as myocardial contusions, incurred at the same time as the neurologic trauma, may manifest themselves and complicate the clinical picture.

Goals for respiratory management of the patient include ensuring adequate oxygen delivery to other organs and maintaining acid–base equilibrium, in addition to achieving optimal lung function and preventing further injury to the lungs if they are being considered for transplantation. Mechanical ventilation is always necessary. In general, the inspired fraction of oxygen should be kept at less than 50%, peak inspiratory pressures less than 30 cm H_2O with tidal volumes of 15 cc/kg, and less than 5 cm H_2O peak end-expiratory pressure (PEEP). Oxygen saturations of at least 95% and pH of 7.4 are also considered standard. In addition, meticulous respiratory care is necessary to minimize colonization of the trachea with pathogenic organisms, as well as the incidence of pneumonia and atelectasis. Excessive levels of PEEP must be avoided to decrease the incidence of barotrauma and aid venous return to the heart.

A variety of other issues more specific to brain-dead organ donors are also important. Hypothermia frequently develops for a variety of reasons, and must be treated aggressively using forced warm-air devices, warming intravenous fluids, and ventilating the lungs with warmed, humidified air. Central temperature monitoring is necessary: the temperature should be kept at or above 35°C. The issue of prophylactic antibiotic use is controversial and center-specific. Coagulopathy, again of multifactorial origin, is also common. While the risk for microvascular thrombosis is high, therapies such as epsilon-aminocaproic acid are not recommended. Defects in coagulation should be treated with replacement therapy guided by deficits in specific factors or platelets. Likewise, endocrine and metabolic disorders should be treated according to frequent laboratory measurements of electrolytes and glucose.

Provision of nutrition to the potential organ donor is also a topic of interest. Significant increases in safe cold ischemia times for livers and other abdominal organs have been achieved with development of University of Wisconsin (UW) solution, providing, among other things, products for continued cellular metabolism. Most organ donors spend at least 2 to 3 days, sometimes in excess of a week, on mechanical ventilation and without nutrition during the process of identification, confirmation of brain death, and preparation for organ procurement. Interestingly, in studies in rats, livers from fasted donors appeared to tolerate long-term preservation better than livers from fed donors, but improved survival was seen in rats fed glucose (40% in drinking water) for 4 days prior to transplant. The investigators proposed that this was due to elevation of liver glycogen levels in the allograft. This would allow for improved capacity for anaerobically derived ATP during the ischemic period and better-maintained hepatocyte viability. With shorter periods of glucose intake, smaller amounts of benefit were seen, but they were still considered to be helpful. If this observation is confirmed in further laboratory investigations, it is possible that once a patient has been declared brain-dead and further neurologic injury is no longer an issue, providing glucose infusions but avoiding hyperglycemia may become common practice.

REFERENCE

1. Schroeder RA, Kuo PC. Organ allocation and donor management. In: Kuo PC, Schroeder RA, Johnson LB, eds. *Clinical management of the transplant patient.* London: Arnold, 2001:201–227.

Chapter 2

Heart Procurement

■ **Jason A. Petrofski, M.D.**
■ **Carmelo A. Milano, M.D.**

Department of Surgery, Duke University Medical
Center, Durham, NC

Step 1. Donor hearts undergo three studies to evaluate graft quality: echocardio-graphy, right heart catheterization, and in older donors, coronary angiography.

Step 2. Upon arrival at the donor hospital, the harvesting surgeon confirms the declaration of brain death and ABO compatibility and size compatibility between the donor and planned recipient.

Step 3. Prepare and drape the donor in a standard sterile fashion from the chest to the thighs.

Step 4. Perform a median sternotomy and spread the sternum with a standard chest retractor.

Step 5. Open and tack up the pericardium, suspending the heart for better expo-sure.

Step 6. Particularly in cases of traumatic death, inspect the heart for any areas of contusion.

Step 7. Palpate the coronary arteries to exclude calcification or plaque. Inspect the right ventricle to ensure normal contractility. Tilt the heart toward the right side to confirm normal contractility of the left ventricular free wall.

Step 8. Avoid extensive retraction of the heart or dissection to prevent arrhyth-mias or hypotension, which may compromise the rest of the multi-organ harvest. Further dissection should take place just before the heart is arrested and harvested.

Step 9. With electrocautery, divide the adventitial attachments between the main pulmonary artery and the ascending aorta.

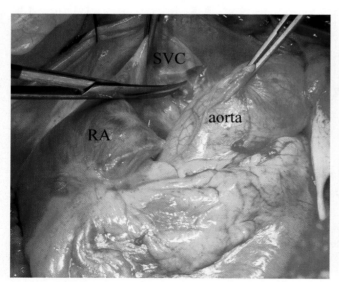

Figure 2-1.

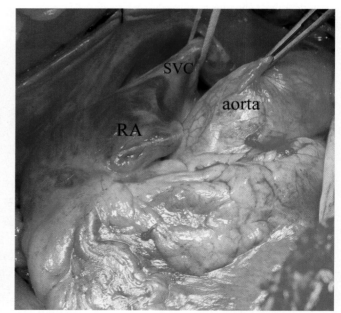

Figure 2-2.

Step 10. Mobilization of superior vena cava. Mobilize the superior vena cava (SVC) to the level of the innominate vein. Encircle the SVC with two ligatures. If the bicaval operative technique will be used, do not use ligatures; the entire SVC is preserved (Figs. 2-1 and 2-2).

Step 11. Mobilization of inferior vena cava. Mobilize the inferior vena cava (IVC) from the pericardial reflection.

Step 12. Separation of right atrium from left. Dissect the interatrial groove (Waterston's groove) to help separate the right atrium and SVC from the left atrium and pulmonary veins.

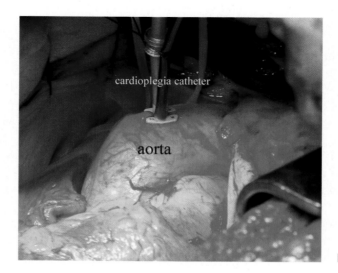

Figure 2-3.

Step 13. Insertion of cannula. Insert a cardioplegia perfusion cannula in the ascending aorta and secure it with a purse-string suture (Fig. 2-3).

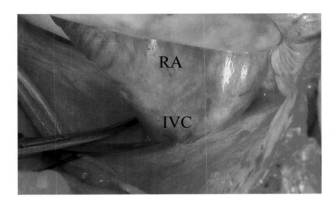

Figure 2-4.

Step 14. Division of IVC. During abdominal organ dissection, keep the heart moistened with a saline-damped sponge. Once all dissection is completed, administer heparin intravenously at 300 U/kg. Divide the inferior vena cava (IVC) just above the diaphragm, allowing blood to drain into the right chest. The SVC may be ligated at this point. After several cardiac cycles, the heart is relatively empty and the ascending aorta can be cross-clamped (Fig. 2-4).

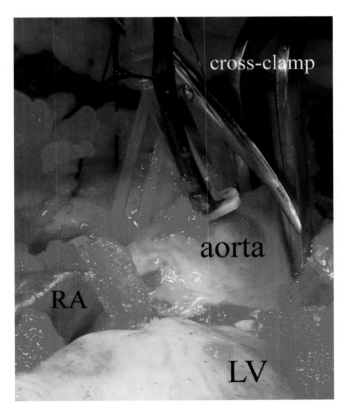

Figure 2-5.

Step 15. Division of aorta. Vent the left atrium by an incision in the left atrial appendage or, if the lungs are not harvested, by an incision into the left pulmonary vein. Deliver cold preservative solution (4°C) to the coronary circulation via the perfusion cannula at a pressure of 150 mm Hg using a pressure bag. The heart is topically cooled with ice-cold saline (4°C). If the standard method of cardiac transplantation is planned, ligate the SVC approximately 2 to 3 cm from the right atrium. If the bicaval operative technique is used, ligate the SVC at the level of the innominate vein. After 1 L cold preservative solution is administered, divide the aorta at the level of the arch. If more aorta is needed, the entire arch can be taken (Fig. 2-5).

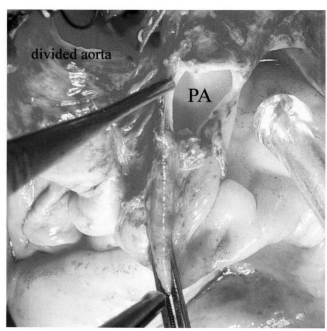

Figure 2-6.

Step 16. Division of pulmonary artery. Divide the pulmonary artery (PA) at its bifurcation. If the lungs are to be procured, leave the left pulmonary artery intact (Fig. 2-6).

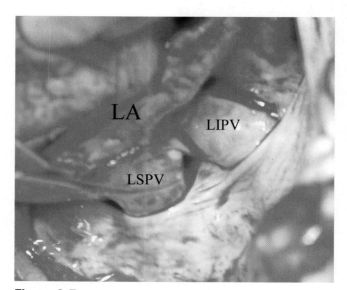

Figure 2-7.

Step 17. Mobilization of the heart. Divide the already ligated SVC. Elevate the heart from the pericardium and divide the pulmonary veins individually at the pericardial reflection (Figs. 2-7 and 2-8A).

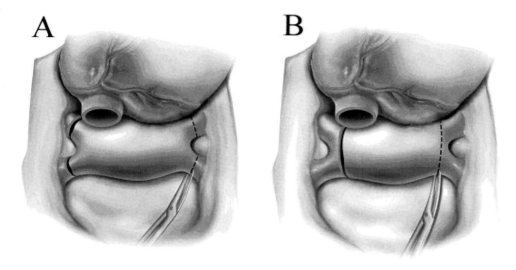

Figure 2-8. Donor organ pulmonary vein division.

Step 18. Mobilization of the heart (2). If the lungs are also being procured, then the donor cardiectomy is modified at several steps. Take care to divide the main pulmonary artery proximal to the bifurcation. Leave the entire bifurcation for the lung grafts. Carefully divide the left atrium, leaving a cuff of left atrial tissue with the right and left pulmonary veins to facilitate the lung transplant. In this setting, divide the left atrium at the midpoint between the coronary sinus and the pulmonary veins (Fig. 2-8B).

Step 19. Preservation of the heart. Remove the heart from the chest and place it into a sterile bag filled with cold preservative. It should be transported in a cooler at 4°C. The bag containing the heart should be carefully labeled with the UNOS donor identification number and the donor blood type.

Chapter 3

Lung Procurement

■ **Matthew G. Hartwig, M.D.**

■ **Shu S. Lin, M.D., Ph.D.**

■ **Sinan A. Simsir, M.D.**

■ **R. Duane Davis, M.D.**

Department of Surgery, Duke University Medical Center, Durham, NC

INTRODUCTION

The lung transplant begins with evaluation of potential donor organs. To limit reperfusion injury, ischemic time needs to be minimized, so all members of the transplant team must be in close contact throughout the procedure. If both the heart and lungs are deemed suitable for procurement, you should always be able to safely remove both of these organs, and the following discussion will assume simultaneous collection of the heart and lungs for transplantation.

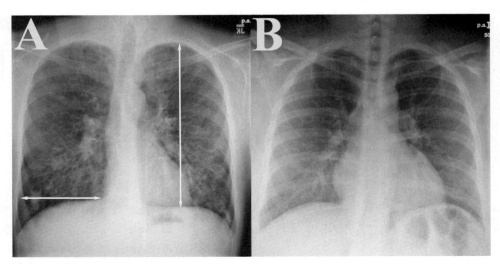

Figure 3-1.

Step 1. Selection of organs. The evaluation of the lungs includes obtaining a thorough medical history of the potential donor. Specific criteria depend on the transplant center, but in general you should focus on the donor's blood type, age, smoking habits, pulmonary diseases, thoracic procedures, and mode of death. After obtaining consent for procurement, give corticosteroids to the donor. Examine the most recent chest radiograph for pathology; it can also be used to help with sizing of the organs. The chest radiographs in Figure 3-1 show (A) a cystic fibrosis recipient with horizontal and vertical measurements and (B) the potential donor without obvious pathology. Atelectasis may not preclude transplantation, but clear consolidation would prevent use of the organs, unless only the contralateral lung were to be used. Also, blood gas analysis should show a minimum PaO_2 of 300 mm Hg on a FiO_2 of 1.0 and peak end-expiratory pressure (PEEP) of 5 cm H_2O just before procurement. When the initial blood gas demonstrates poor oxygenation, perform therapeutic bronchoscopy before repeating the blood gas in order to remove secretions, recruit atelectactic lung segments, and ventilate with appropriate tidal volumes. Peak inspiratory pressure should be less than 30 cm H_2O.

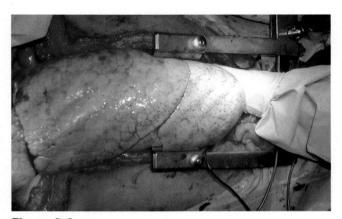

Figure 3-2.

Step 2. Lung inspection. Direct evaluation of the lungs before procurement includes flexible bronchoscopy to evaluate the airways. Remove easily cleared secretions. Thick, purulent secretions or obvious evidence of extensive aspiration is usually exclusionary, unless only one lung is affected and the contralateral lung is to be procured. Manually inspect the lung parenchyma, looking for nodules, edema, or emphysematous changes. Excise suspicious findings and send them for pathologic analysis to rule out malignancy. By using alveolar recruitment maneuvers, you can also differentiate between atelectasis and consolidation of the parenchyma at this time. Assess the elastic recoil of the lungs one side at a time. First bring the entire lung out of the chest cavity and then inflate the lungs manually with bagged breaths. Then allow the lungs to spontaneously deflate by temporarily disconnecting the endotracheal tube from the ventilator. As illustrated in Figure 3-2, once the lung is gently displaced out of the thoracic cavity, the donor lungs are three-quarters inflated to remove atelectasis and evaluate lung compliance. Repeat the same maneuver on the contralateral side. Lungs with adequate compliance should rapidly deflate following disconnection from the ventilator.

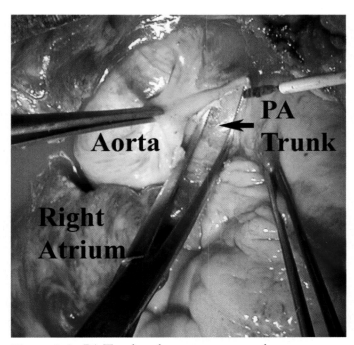

Figure 3-3. PA Trunk, pulmonary artery trunk.

Step 3. Preparation for procurement. After evaluation of the donor lungs is completed, the surgical procurement can begin. The patient has already been prepared and draped in the standard fashion and a midline sternotomy performed for the manual inspection of the lungs. Open the pericardium and place stay sutures to expose its contents. Begin dissection. Expose the great vessels (Fig. 3-3).

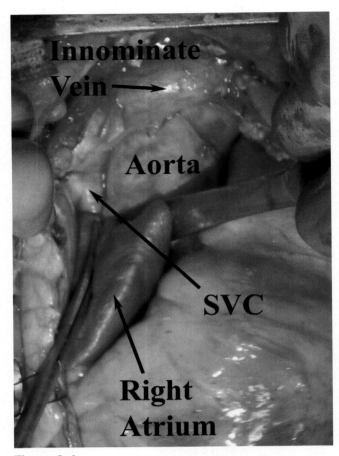

Figure 3-4.

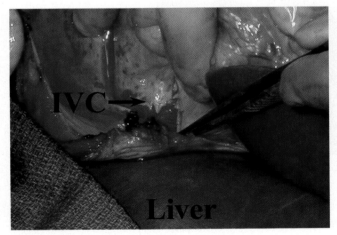

Figure 3-5.

Step 4. Exposure of the superior vena cava and inferior vena cava. Expose the superior vena cava (SVC) by dissecting between the SVC and the aorta (Fig. 3-4). The inferior vena cava (IVC) should be well exposed above and below the diaphragm to ensure adequate vessel length for the abdominal and cardiac transplant teams (Fig. 3-5). Encircle both the SVC and the IVC with silk sutures. Temporary hemodynamic instability commonly occurs, but this can be decreased by placing the donor in the Trendelenburg position before carrying out these maneuvers.

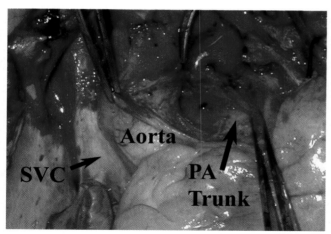

Figure 3-6.

Step 5. Development of plane between aorta and right pulmonary artery.
Dissect the right pulmonary artery from the SVC and ascending aorta (Fig. 3-6).
Avoid injuring the right pulmonary artery as it passes laterally to the SVC, as this
would need to be repaired before transplantation. The azygous vein can be ligated
at this time.

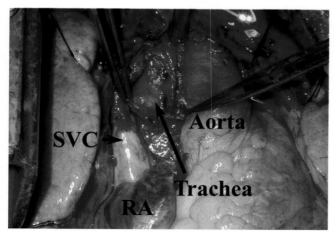

Figure 3-7.

Step 6. Identifying the trachea. Complete the dissection by exposing the aor-
topulmonary window for placement of the aortic cross-clamp and the trachea for
future stapling. Locate the trachea by incising the posterior pericardium after gently retracting the SVC laterally and the aorta medially (Fig. 3-7). It can be visualized cephalad to the right atrium (RA) and posterior to the SVC and aorta.

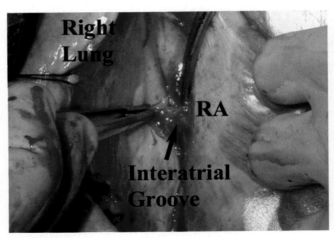

Figure 3-8.

Step 7. Preparation for left atrial cuff. Dissecting the interatrial groove at this time facilitates subsequent creation of the left atrial cuff. This also allows better visualization of the right pulmonary veins (Fig. 3-8).

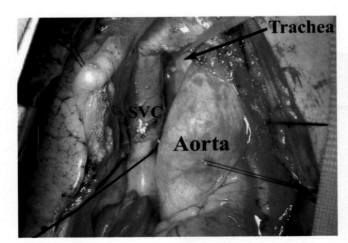

Figure 3-9.

Step 8. Isolating the trachea. Umbilical tape can be used to encircle the trachea after the plane is developed manually. Dissection of the great vessels is now complete for cannulization of the aorta and pulmonary trunk (Fig. 3-9).

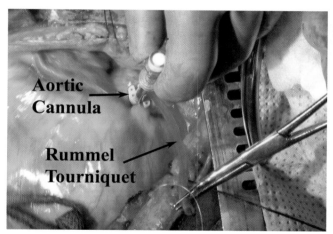

Figure 3-10.

Step 9. Cannulization of ascending aorta. Before placement of the aortic and pulmonary artery cannulas, the patient should be fully heparinized (more than 400 U/kg). Cannulate the ascending aorta for standard antegrade cardioplegia. Secure the cannula using a 4-0 prolene mattress or purse-string suture and a Rummel tourniquet (Fig. 3-10).

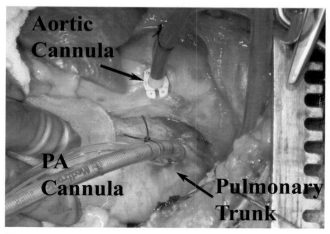

Figure 3-11.

Step 10. Cannulization of pulmonary artery. Next, the pulmonary artery (PA) cannula is placed in a similar fashion as the aortic cannula (Fig. 3-11). The placement should be comfortably distal to the pulmonary valve, but proximal enough to ensure equal perfusion through both pulmonary arteries. Also, ensure that the bent tip of the 6.5-mm curved cannula is directed toward the bifurcation.

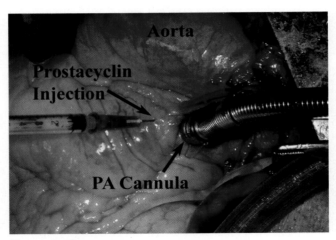

Figure 3-12.

Step 11. Injection of pulmonary vasodilator. After placing the cannulas, give a 500-μg bolus dose of prostacyclin directly into the pulmonary trunk near the pulmonary artery cannula (PA) insertion site (Fig. 3-12).

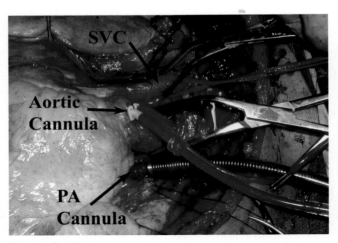

Figure 3-13.

Step 12. Positioning vascular clamps. Position the SVC and aortic clamps as shown for vascular occlusion immediately before perfusion of the heart–lung bloc with low-potassium dextran preservation solution (Fig. 3-13).

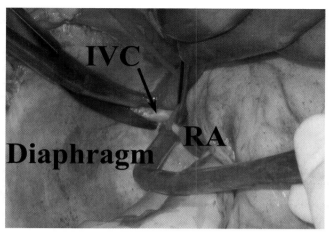

Figure 3-14.

Step 13. Dividing the IVC. Immediately after infusion of the prostacyclin, ligate the SVC or occlude it using a vascular clamp and divide the IVC, allowing decompression of the right side of the heart (Fig. 3-14). Divide the IVC above the pericardial reflection to provide an adequate cuff for both the liver and heart implantations.

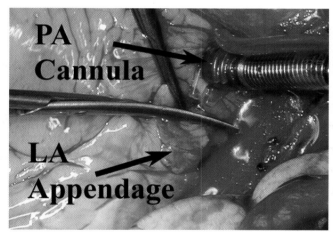

Figure 3-15.

Step 14. Decompression of left side of the heart. Decompress the left side of the heart with a sizable left atrial (LA) appendage incision. Then cross-clamp the aorta and infuse the cardioplegia solution through the aortic cannula. Even if the heart is not to be procured, aortic cross-clamping prevents bronchial artery flow and should be performed at this point. At the same time, infuse Perfadex® or Celsior® preservation solution through the pulmonary artery cannula. Incise the left atrial appendage, preventing distention of the left cardiac chambers (Fig. 3-15). Flush 50 mL/kg of perfusate through the pulmonary arteries. The same solution can be used for cardiac preservation following cardioplegia. Avoid distending the heart with preservation solution.

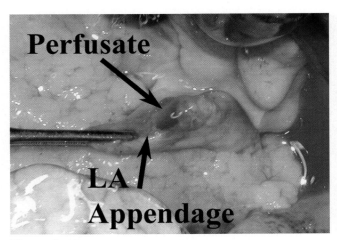

Figure 3-16.

Step 15. Perfusion of organs. When perfusate flow begins, bathe the thoracic cavity in iced saline solution. Assess biventricular filling by directly palpating the heart. Note exsanguination and subsequent flow of clear fluid from the left atrial appendage (Fig. 3-16). After adequate preservation, prepare for the removal of the heart. Again, with appropriate procurement techniques, the heart and lung teams should both be able to remove suitable organs.

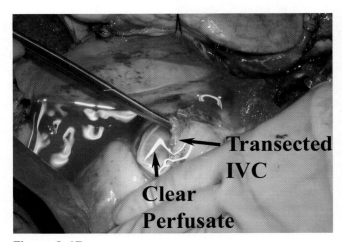

Figure 3-17.

Step 16. Mobilization of IVC. Circumferentially free the IVC and mobilize it to the right atrium. Again, note clear perfusate, this time from the divided IVC (Fig. 3-17).

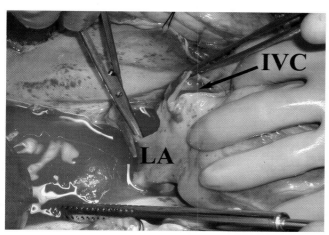

Figure 3-18.

Step 17. Preparation of left atrial cuff. Retract the heart to the right and begin a left atriotomy between the coronary sinus and the left pulmonary veins. Further develop the interatrial groove on the right to ensure adequate atrial cuff size. Extend the initial atriotomy inferiorly and superiorly using scissors, while being mindful of the left pulmonary veins. The surgeon on the left side of the table typically has the optimal view of the right pulmonary vein orifices and should finish creating the atrial cuff while directly visualizing the right venous orifices. In Figure 3-18, the procuring surgeon carefully creates the atrial cuff by extending the initial atriotomy.

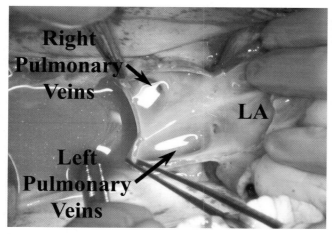

Figure 3-19.

Step 18. Division of left atrium. The pulmonary veins are now exposed and the remaining left atrium can be divided safely. Enough cuff width should be available for proper suturing of the pulmonary vein anastomosis (Fig. 3-19).

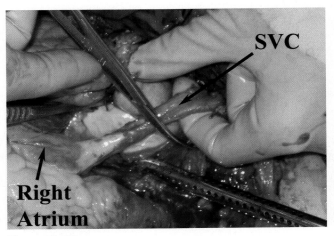

Figure 3-20.

Step 19. Division of SVC. Divide the SVC proximal to the silk ligature, using scissors (Fig. 3-20). If a vascular clamp is in position, you can maximize the length of SVC taken by repositioning the clamp distally at this time.

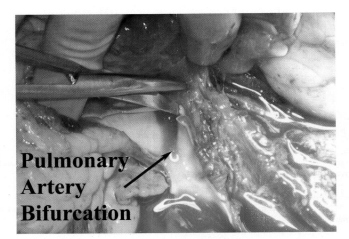

Figure 3-21.

Step 20. Transection of main pulmonary artery. Remove the aortic clamp and mobilize an adequate length of aorta before dividing it. Transect the main pulmonary artery at its bifurcation after removing the pulmonary artery cannula; this provides an adequate conduit for both heart and lung transplant teams (Fig. 3-21).

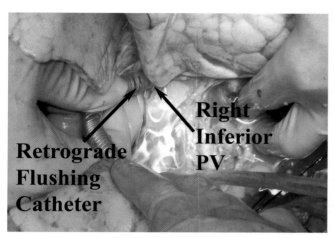

Figure 3-22.

Step 21. Retrograde pulmonary flushing. Remove the heart from the field. After the heart is passed off the table, perform retrograde flushing of the lungs. Using the previously removed pulmonary artery cannula, infuse each of the four pulmonary veins with a minimum of 250 to 500 mL (Fig. 3-22). Continue retrograde flushing until clear perfusate is noted eluting from the pulmonary artery.

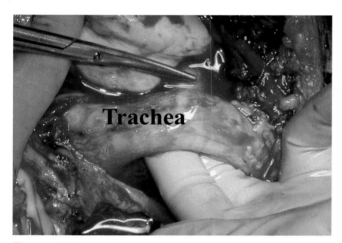

Figure 3-23.

Step 22. Development of plane between trachea and esophagus. Divide the inferior pulmonary ligaments and posterior attachments. Mobilize the trachea to three cartilaginous rings proximal to the carina (Fig. 3-23).

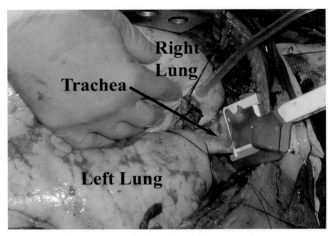

Figure 3-24.

Step 23. Stapling the trachea. Before stapling the trachea, ask the anesthesia team to reposition the endotracheal tube more proximally and provide several bagged breaths. This step eliminates residual atelectasis and allows the lungs to deflate to approximately two-thirds vital capacity. Staple the trachea with the TA-30 stapler two or three rings above the carina, while avoiding overinflation of the lungs. Both lungs pictured in Figure 3-24 are partially inflated. Coordination with the anesthesiology team is critical during this portion of the case.

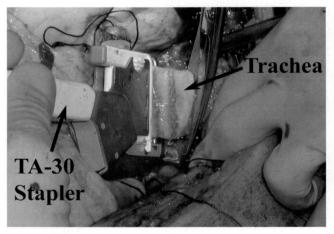

Figure 3-25.

Step 24. Transection of trachea. Place a second row of staples immediately proximal, and divide the trachea between the two staple lines with a scalpel or scissors (Fig. 3-25). The proximal staples prevent the endotracheal contents from spilling into the sterile thoracic cavity.

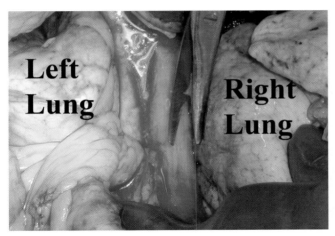

Figure 3-26.

Step 25. Removal of the lungs. Use heavy scissors to swiftly divide the remaining posterior mediastinal tissues inferiorly and superiorly, completely freeing the lungs for removal (Fig. 3-26). Take care not to perforate either the trachea or esophagus to avoid contaminating the field and deflating the lungs. An alternative method requires stapling the proximal and distal thoracic esophagus with a GIA stapler, with the remaining dissection occurring between the esophagus and the spine and subsequent removal of the lungs en bloc with the esophagus (not shown).

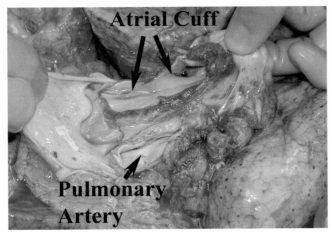

Figure 3-27.

Step 26. Inspection of lungs. Immediate back-table examination of the lungs ensures no damage has been done to the organs. Figure 3-27 illustrates the initial view of the pulmonary grafts after removal from the donor but before excess tissue is removed.

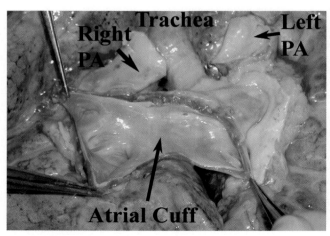

Figure 3-28.

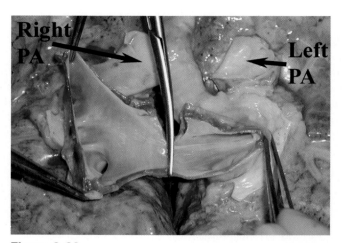

Figure 3-29.

Step 27. Separation of left atrial cuffs. At this point, place the lungs in a bag if they will travel together; if they are going to separate institutions, divide them now. In either scenario, divide the lungs by incising the posterior pericardium, the left atrium between the two sets of veins, and the main pulmonary artery at its bifurcation. In Figure 3-28, the atrial cuff is exposed, showing the right and left inferior and superior vein orifices. Figure 3-29 illustrates the division of the atrial cuff between the right and left pulmonary veins with scissors. If being separated prior to travel, the left bronchus can be transected between staples just distal to the carina to maintain its inflation pressure for transport.

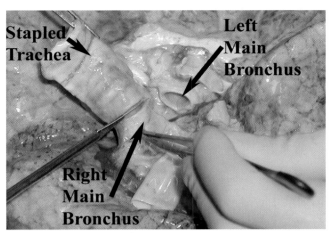

Figure 3-30.

Step 28. Preparation for implantation. When they arrive at the transplanting institution, prepare the grafts for implantation. This primarily involves dividing the main bronchus for each lung approximately two rings proximal to the upper lobe take-off. In Figure 3-30, the right main bronchus is being divided with a scalpel proximal to the take-off of the right superior bronchus. The left main bronchus has already been divided. Minimize dissection along the length of the bronchus. Inspect the pulmonary arteries to their first branches for injury. Also evaluate the arteries and atrial cuff for residual pericardial attachments; remove them at this time because if retained, they may lead to kinking and blood flow occlusion after the anastomosis is completed. Samples of donor bronchus for microbiologic testing can also be taken at this time.

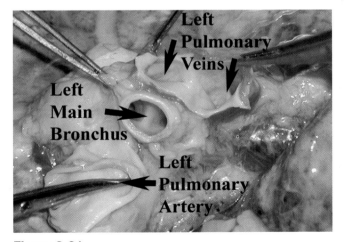

Figure 3-31.

Step 29. Preparation for implantation (2). Following completion of the dissection, the three major structures to be anastomosed to the recipient are depicted in Figure 3-31. The graft is now ready for implantation as a single graft or bilateral sequential single lung transplants.

Chapter 4

Liver, Kidney, and Pancreas Procurement

■ **Carlos E. Marroquin, M.D.**
■ **Paul C. Kuo, M.D.**

Department of Surgery, Duke University Medical Center, Durham, NC

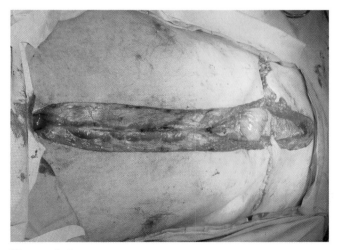

Figure 4-1.

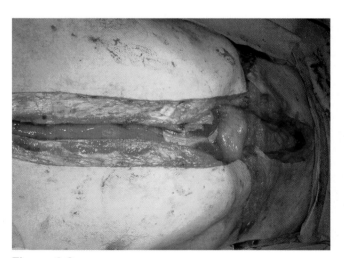

Figure 4-2.

Step 1. Positioning and approach. With the donor positioned with arms extended, make a midline incision from the suprasternal notch to the pubis (Fig. 4-1).

Step 2. Approach. If additional exposure is required, a transverse incision can be made to form a cruciate incision (Fig. 4-2).

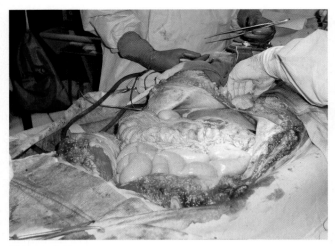

Figure 4-3.

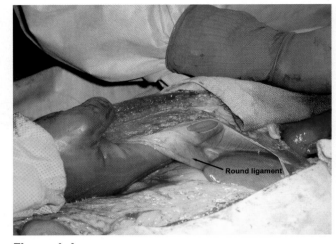

Figure 4-4.

Step 3. Approach (2). Figure 4-3 shows exposure with combined midline and cruciate incisions.

Step 4. Exploration of abdomen. Divide the round ligament. Explore the abdomen for hepatic arterial anomalies, mass lesions, and arterial aneurysmal disease. Place a retractor (Fig. 4-4).

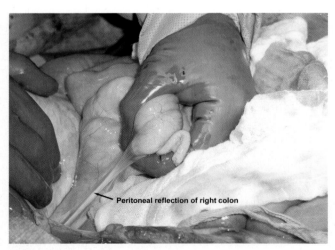

Figure 4-5.

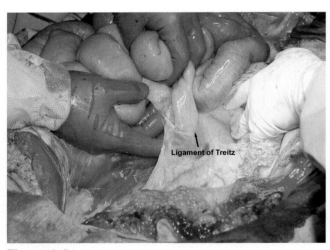

Figure 4-6.

Step 5. Mobilization of right colon. Mobilize the right colon along the peritoneal reflection. Fully mobilize the right colon and small bowel mesentery to the level of the ligament of Treitz. Expose Gerota's fascia of the right kidney anteriorly and posteriorly to allow contact with topical slush (Fig. 4-5).

Step 6. Mobilization of right colon (2). Complete mobilization of the right colon and small bowel mesentery (Fig. 4-6).

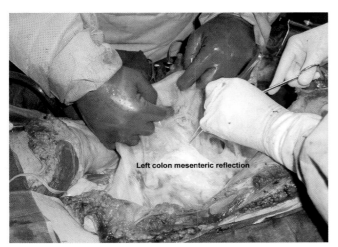

Figure 4-7.

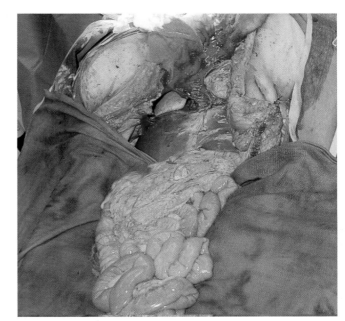

Figure 4-8.

Step 7. Mobilization of left colon. Mobilize the left colon similarly to expose Gerota's fascia surrounding the left kidney (Fig. 4-7).

Step 8. Exposure of inferior vena cava (IVC) and aorta. Wrapping the intestines can aid in exposure of the IVC and aorta (Fig. 4-8).

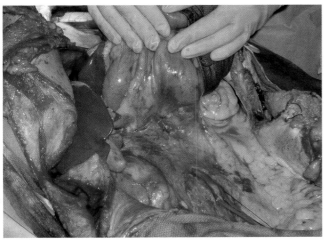

Figure 4-9.

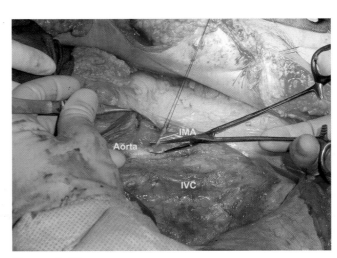

Figure 4-10.

Step 9. Exposure of IVC and aorta. Figure 4-9 shows exposure of the IVC and aorta.

Step 10. Division of inferior mesenteric artery. Ligate and divide the inferior mesenteric artery (Fig. 4-10).

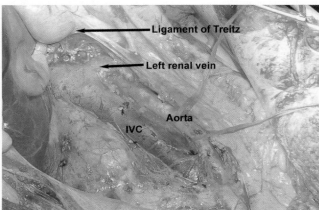

Figure 4-11.

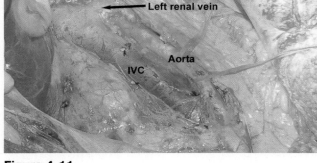

Figure 4-12.

Step 11. Exposure of vena cava and aorta. Expose the vena cava and aorta and encircle them with vascular tapes. Identify the left renal vein (Fig. 4-11).

Step 12. Exposure of superior mesenteric artery. Immediately superior to the left renal vein, expose the superior mesenteric artery through the ganglial tissue at its juncture with the aorta. Return the bowel to normal position (Fig. 4-12).

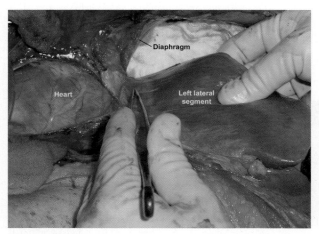

Figure 4-13.

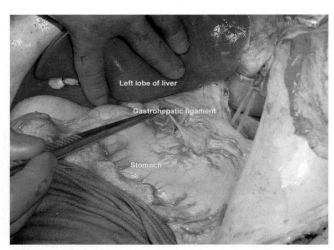

Figure 4-14.

Step 13. Division of left triangular ligament. Figure 4-13 shows division of the left triangular ligament.

Step 14. Exposure of caudate lobe. Divide the gastrohepatic ligament to expose the caudate lobe. Take care to identify and preserve an accessory or replaced left hepatic artery. If present, dissect the replaced artery retrograde along the lesser curvature of the stomach to its junction with the left gastric artery (Fig. 4-14). Inspect the porta hepatis and palpate it for the left, right, and main proper hepatic arteries. Perform a Kocher maneuver to expose the retropancreatic inferior vena cava. An accessory or replaced right hepatic artery can be palpated along its course from the superior mesenteric artery posterior to the pancreas to a posterior position in the hilum. Mobilize the right lobe of the liver, if desired.

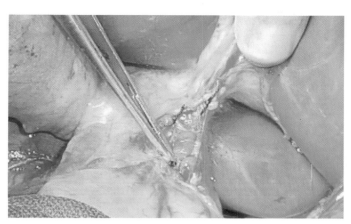

Figure 4-15.

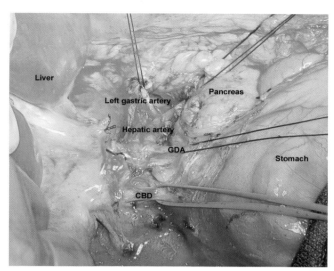

Figure 4-16.

Step 15. Exposure of common hepatic artery. Expose the common hepatic artery along the superior edge of the pancreas, beginning under the "Starzlian" lymph node at the junction of the pancreas and porta hepatis (Fig. 4-15).

Step 16. Identification of left gastric and splenic arteries. Trace the proper and common hepatic artery back to the level of the celiac axis, where the left gastric and splenic arteries can be identified. Also identify the gastroduodenal artery during this dissection (Fig. 4-16).

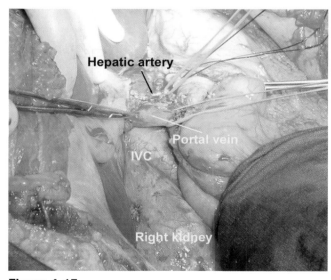

Figure 4-17.

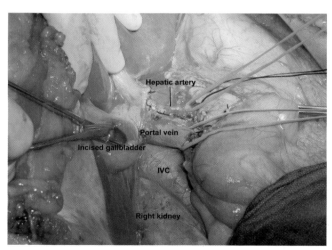

Figure 4-18.

Step 17. Division of common bile duct. Ligate and divide the gastroduodenal artery to expose the portal vein. Dissect the portal vein away from surrounding adventitial tissue. Ligate the distal common bile duct close to the pancreas and divide the duct (Fig. 4-17).

Step 18. Flushing gallbladder. Incise the gallbladder and flush it with cold saline. Note clear effluent from the proximal end of the divided common bile duct (Fig. 4-18).

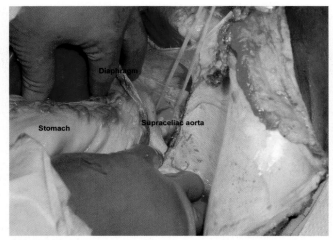

Figure 4-19.

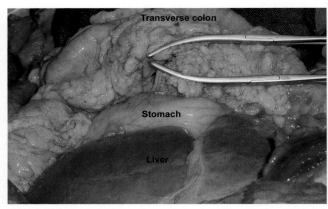

Figure 4-20.

Step 19. Exposure of supraceliac aorta. Expose the supraceliac aorta through the crura of the diaphragm. Sufficient exposure should be available for emergent aortic cross-clamping, if necessary (Fig. 4-19).

Step 20. Division of omental vessels. Enter the lesser sac. Clamp, divide, and ligate the omental vessels between the greater curve of the stomach and the transverse colon (Fig. 4-20).

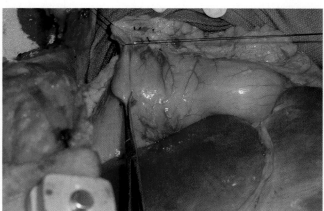

Figure 4-21.

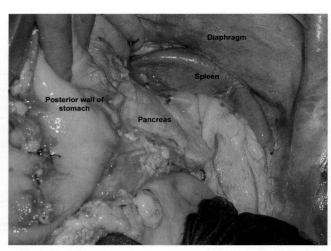

Figure 4-22.

Step 21. Division of short gastric vessels. Ligate and divide the short gastric vessels (Fig. 4-21).

Step 22. Visualization of spleen. Divide adhesions between the anterior surface of the pancreas and the posterior wall of the stomach using electrocautery. The entire anterior surface of the spleen can now be visualized (Fig. 4-22).

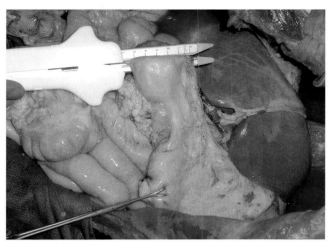

Figure 4-23.

Step 23. Division of duodenum. Divide the duodenum immediately distal to the pylorus (Fig. 4-23). The stomach may be packed away. (This may also be performed following flushing of organs.)

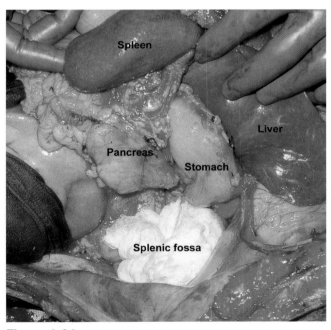

Figure 4-24.

Step 24. Mobilization of spleen and pancreas. Fully mobilize the spleen and tail of pancreas to the level of the splenic artery and the lateral margin of the aorta. Ligate and divide the lienocolic ligaments. The head of the pancreas should already have been mobilized with the Kocher maneuver (Fig. 4-24). Incise the ligament of Treitz sufficiently to be able to derotate the small bowel under the small bowel mesentery.

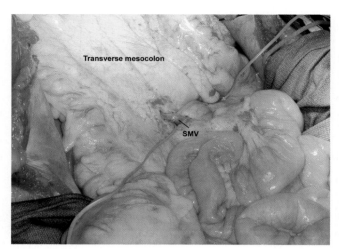

Figure 4-25.

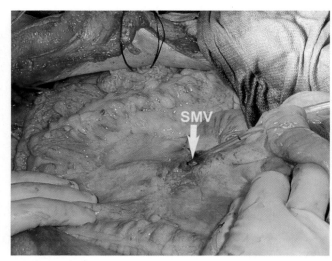

Figure 4-26.

Step 25. Cannulation of splanchnic venous circulation. Expose the superior mesenteric vein at the base of the transverse colon for cannulation of the splanchnic venous circulation. Alternative sites for cannulation include the inferior mesenteric vein or portal vein. This can be omitted in an emergency (Fig. 4-25).

Step 26. Insertion of splanchnic venous cannula. Following full heparinization, insert and secure the splanchnic venous cannula (Fig. 4-26).

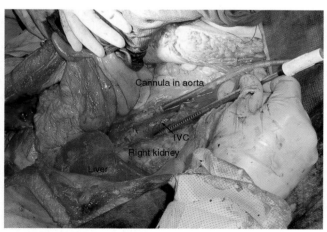

Figure 4-27.

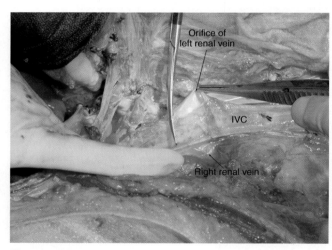

Figure 4-28.

Step 27. Insertion and securing of aortic and vena caval cannulas. After the aortic and vena caval cannulas are inserted and secured, clamp the supraceliac aorta in conjunction with the thoracic procurement teams (Fig. 4-27). Flush the abdominal organs with preservation solution through the aortic and mesenteric cannulas. Apply iced slush solution to achieve topical cooling. Vent effluent through the vena caval cannula. Following complete removal of the thoracic organs, begin the procedure for retrieval of the liver, pancreas, and renal organs. The pancreas is removed first.

Step 28. Division of left renal vein. Divide the left renal vein at its entrance into the IVC. Then divide the IVC above the entry of the renal veins (Fig. 4-28).

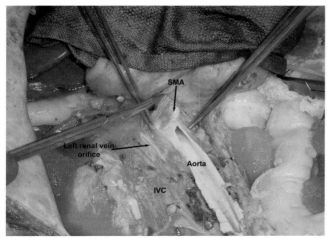

Figure 4-29.

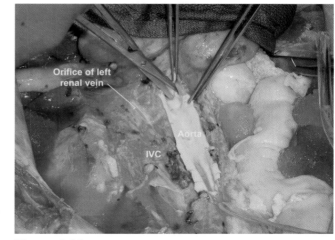

Figure 4-30.

Step 29. Division of aorta and superior mesenteric artery. Divide the aorta anteriorly and identify the orifices of the renal arteries from within the aorta. Divide the superior mesenteric artery at the junction with the aorta (Fig. 4-29).

Step 30. Transection of aorta. Transect the aorta below the superior mesenteric artery junction to avoid injuring the renal vessels (Fig. 4-30).

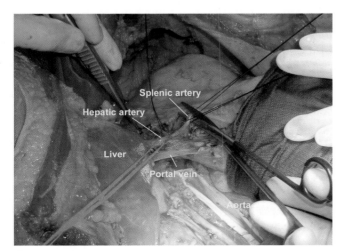

Figure 4-31.

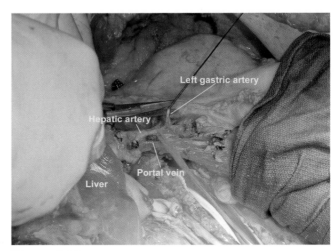

Figure 4-32.

Step 31. Division of splenic artery. (Fig. 4-31)

Step 32. Division of left gastric artery. (Fig. 4-32)

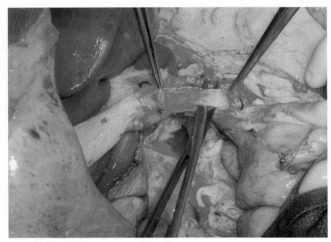

Figure 4-33.

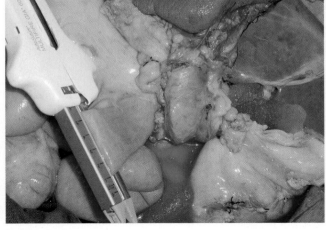

Figure 4-34.

Step 33. Division of portal vein. Divide the portal vein at the level of the coronary vein (Fig. 4-33).

Step 34. Division of jejunum. Derotate the small bowel under the mesentery of the transverse colon. Divide the jejunum approximately 10 cm distal to the ligament of Treitz (Fig. 4-34).

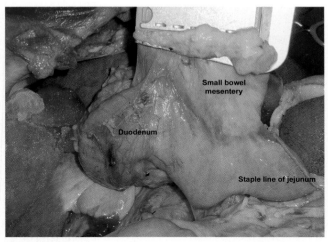

Figure 4-35.

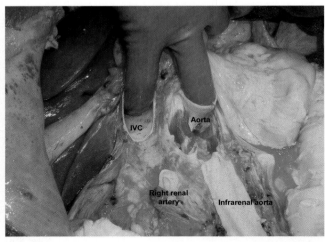

Figure 4-36.

Step 35. Division of small bowel mesentery. Divide the small bowel mesentery using serial fires of a vascular stapler. Leave a generous margin of small bowel mesentery attached to the pancreas to avoid injury to the superior mesenteric artery and vein (Fig. 4-35). Remove the pancreas with the attached spleen, and attention is directed to the liver.

Step 36. Mobilization of liver. Incise the diaphragm to fully mobilize the right lobe of the liver. Divide the supraceliac aorta at the level of the cross-clamp. Insert fingers into the aorta and cava from below to lift the liver (Fig. 4-36). Remove the liver by cutting through the paraspinous muscles. Next, focus attention on the kidneys.

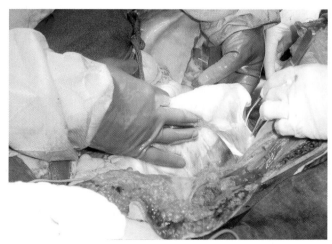

Figure 4-37.

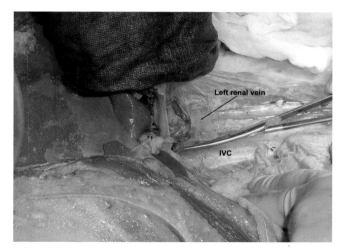

Figure 4-38.

Step 37. Mobilization of kidney and adrenal gland. Fully mobilize the left kidney and adrenal gland, taking care to preserve Gerota's fascia. Make an opening in the left colonic mesentery to transfer the left kidney medially (Fig. 4-37).

Step 38. Division of left renal vein. Divide the left renal vein at the junction with the IVC (Fig. 4-38).

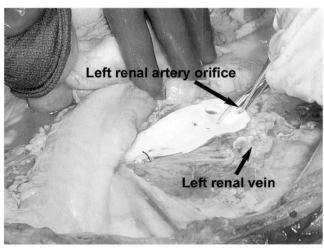

Figure 4-39.

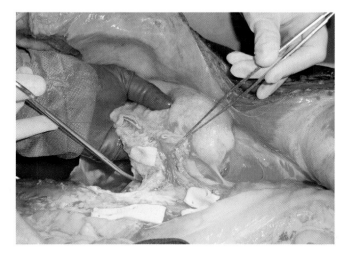

Figure 4-40.

Step 39. Identification of left renal artery orifice. Identify the left renal artery orifice from within the divided aorta (Fig. 4-39).

Step 40. Removal of left kidney. Remove the left kidney with a long segment of ureter divided at the level of the common iliac vessels (Fig. 4-40).

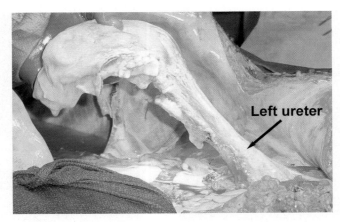

Figure 4-41.

Step 41. Removal of left kidney (2). Figure 4-41 shows a long ureter.

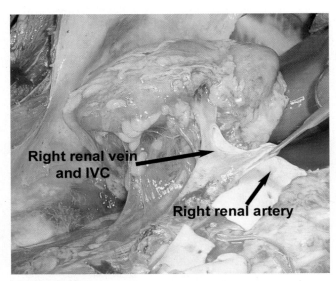

Figure 4-42.

Step 42. Removal of right kidney. Direct attention to the right kidney, which is fully mobilized with an accompanying arterial patch, segment of IVC, and ureter (Fig. 4-42).

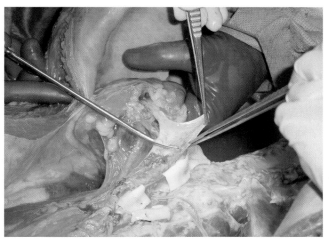

Figure 4-43.

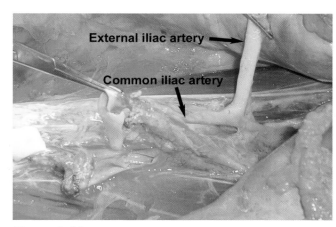

Figure 4-44.

Step 43. Removal of right kidney (2). (Fig. 4-43)

Step 44. Procurement of arteries. Procure long segments of common, external, and internal iliac artery to accompany the liver and pancreas (Fig. 4-44).

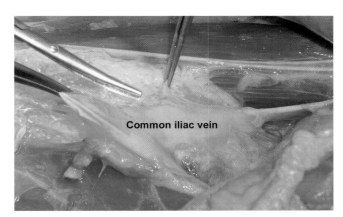

Figure 4-45.

Step 45. Procurement of arteries (2). Procure long segments of common, external, and internal iliac artery to accompany the liver and pancreas (Fig. 4-45). Close the incision.

Section II

Heart Transplantation

Chapter 5

Orthotopic Heart Transplantation

■ **Jason A. Petrofski, M.D.**
■ **Carmelo A. Milano, M.D.**

Department of Surgery, Duke University Medical Center, Durham, NC

INTRODUCTION

Heart transplantation has evolved from an experimental procedure to a commonly performed therapy for end-stage heart failure. The operative technique has been modified minimally from the original technique first described by Lower and Shumway in 1960. The standard technique consists of four anastomoses: the left atrium, right atrium, pulmonary artery, and aorta. Since 1967 this technique has been used in the vast majority of the 50,000 heart transplants performed worldwide.

An alternative bicaval anastomotic technique, introduced in the mid-1990s, consists of five anastomoses: the left atrium, inferior vena cava (IVC), superior vena cava (SVC), pulmonary artery, and aorta. The bicaval technique helps preserve normal atrial anatomy and has been reported to improve atrial contractility, sinus node function, and atrioventricular valve function. At our institution, therefore, the bicaval technique is the procedure of choice. The standard technique is still used in select recipients, particularly those who have extensive scarring from previous operations. In this setting, the standard technique reduces preimplantation dissection.

This chapter describes the steps of orthotopic heart transplantation: donor organ procurement, recipient preparation and cardiectomy, donor organ preparation, and implantation. Both the standard and bicaval techniques are described.

RECIPIENT PREPARATION AND CARDIECTOMY

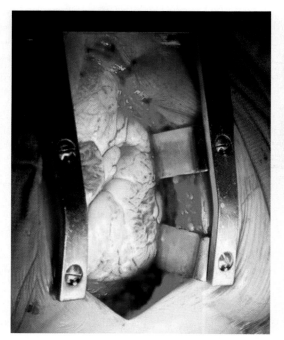

Figure 5-1.

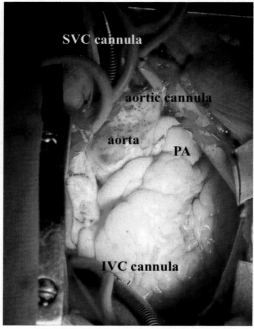

Figure 5-2.

Step 1. Recipient preparation. When the recipient arrives in the operating room, a pulmonary artery catheter is placed and anesthesia is induced. In addition, a femoral arterial line is placed for monitoring and emergency cardiopulmonary bypass cannulation. Once intubated, the recipient is prepared and draped in standard surgical fashion and a median sternotomy is performed (Fig. 5-1).

Step 2. Aortic cannulation. After systemic heparinization, cannulation for cardiopulmonary bypass is performed. Place a double purse-string suture as far distally as possible in the ascending aorta. Insert an aortic cannula and secure it with the purse-string sutures.

Step 3. Venous cannulation. Place purse-string sutures in the SVC and the IVC and place right-angled cannulas for venous drainage (Fig. 5-2).

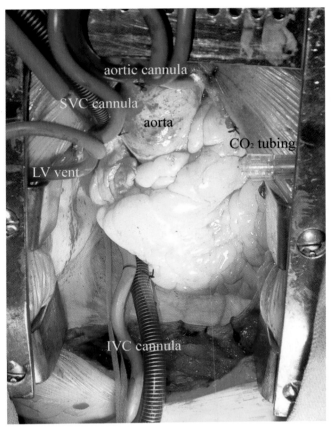

Figure 5-3.

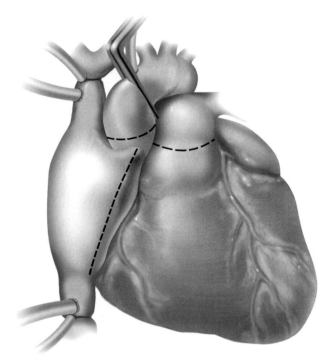

Figure 5-4.

Step 4. Vent the left ventricle. Place a left ventricular vent via the right superior pulmonary vein and secure it with a purse-string suture.

Step 5. CO_2 flooding. Place tubing for CO_2 flooding of the surgical field to reduce the risk of air embolism. CO_2 dissolves more readily in blood and displaces nitrogen.

Step 6. Caval tapes. Place umbilical tape snares around both vena cavae, and complete cardiopulmonary bypass is achieved (Fig. 5-3).

Step 7. Separation of aorta and PA. Using electrocautery, divide the adventitial attachments between the aorta and pulmonary artery. Completely separate the aorta from the main, left, and right pulmonary arteries.

Step 8. Cross-clamp. Cross-clamp the ascending aorta just proximal to the arterial cannula. Figure 5-4 shows the initial lines of transection for the recipient cardiectomy.

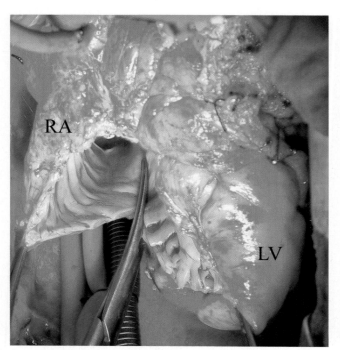

Figure 5-5.

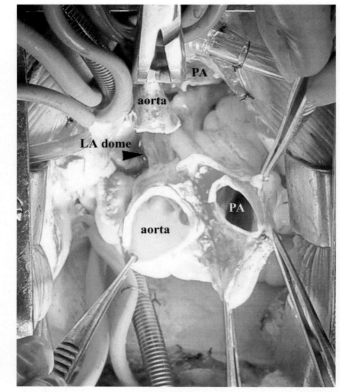

Figure 5-6.

Step 9. Right atrial cuff preparation. Divide the right atrium near the atrioventricular groove. Extend this incision inferiorly, leaving a right atrial cuff for the donor right atrium anastomosis for standard implantation. If using the bicaval technique, further prepare the right atrial cuff as described in Step 12 (Fig. 5-5).

Step 10. Division of aorta and pulmonary artery. Divide both the aorta and the pulmonary artery at the level of the commissures of their respective valves (Fig. 5-6).

Step 11. Left atrial cuff preparation. Transect the left atrium starting at the interatrial septum and continuing around the mitral valve at the level of the atrioventricular groove. Leave a left atrial cuff for donor organ anastomosis.

Step 12. Preparation for bicaval implantation. Excise the native heart at the level of the atrioventricular groove, leaving conjoined right and left atrial cuffs (Fig. 5-7A). For the standard technique, intact right and left atrial cuffs are used and no further dissection is required. For bicaval implantation, dissect the interatrial groove. Separate the right and left atrial cuffs. Trim the left atrial cuff and remove the remnants of the coronary sinus and left atrial appendage (Fig. 5-7B). Trim the right atrial cuff to yield individual SVC and IVC cuffs (Figs. 5-7C and 5-8).

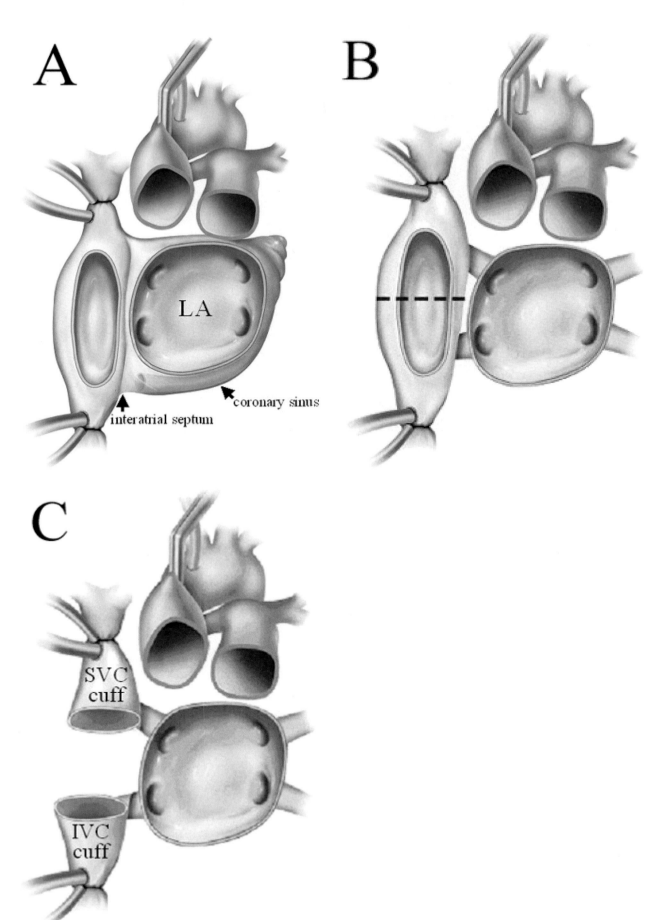

A

LA

interatrial septum

coronary sinus

B

C

SVC
cuff

IVC
cuff

Figure 5-7.

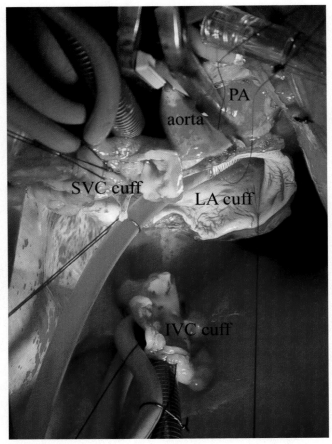

Figure 5-8.

DONOR ORGAN PREPARATION

Step 1. Donor heart preservation. Remove the heart from the transport cooler and place it in a basin of cold saline (2° to 4°).

Step 2. Left atrium preparation. Open the posterior wall of the left atrium by dividing the tissue linking the pulmonary veins (Fig. 5-9). Connecting the pulmonary vein orifice in this manner results in a circular cuff.

Step 3. Examination of interatrial septum. Inspect the interatrial septum for atrial septal defects. In approximately 10% of cases, a patent foramen ovale is present and can be closed with simple sutures.

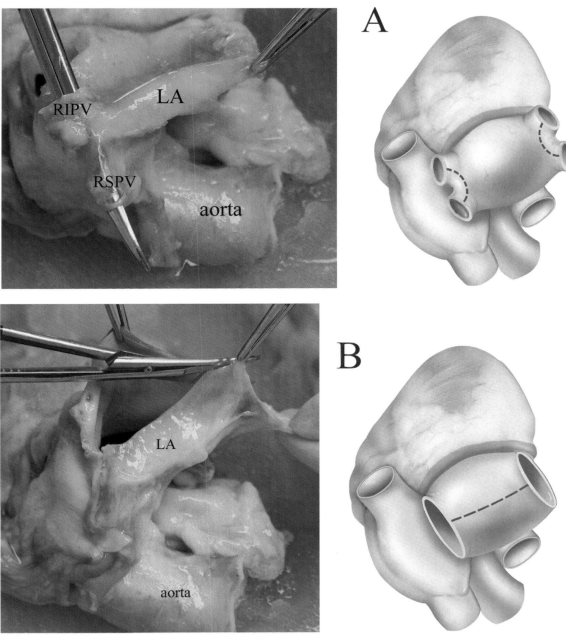

Figure 5-9.

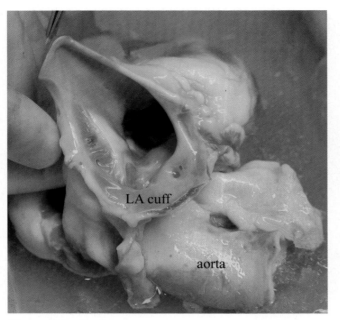

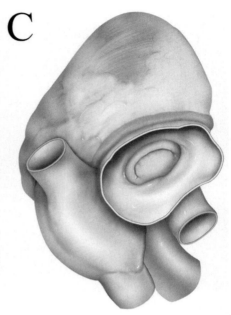

Figure 5-9. *Continued*

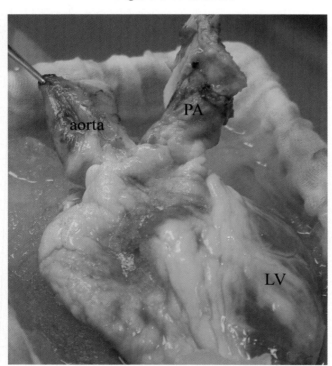

Figure 5-10.

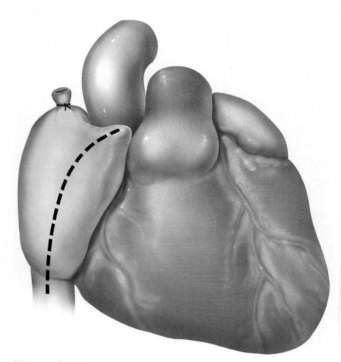

Figure 5-11.

Step 4. Division of adventitial attachments. Using sharp dissection, divide the adventitial attachments between the aorta and pulmonary artery (Fig. 5-10).

Step 5. Preparation for standard implantation technique. For the standard technique of orthotopic heart transplant, open the donor right atrium with a curvilinear incision extending from the IVC orifice through the right atrial appendage. This incision avoids the junction between the SVC and the right atrium, where the sinoatrial node is located. Tie off or oversew the SVC in the donor heart (Fig. 5-11). For the bicaval technique, in which the donor SVC and IVC are anastomosed directly to the recipient SVC and IVC, respectively, the donor right atrium is not opened.

IMPLANTATION PROCEDURE

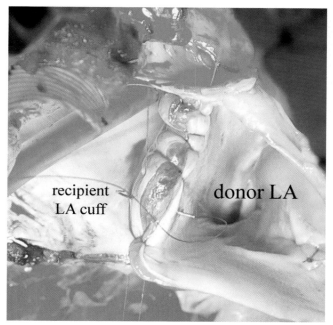

Figure 5-12.

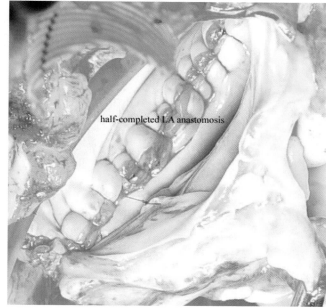

Figure 5-13.

Step 1. Left atrial anastomosis. Sew the recipient left atrial cuff to the donor left atrial remnant with running 3-0 Prolene. Place the first stitches at the level of the recipient's left superior pulmonary vein and near the base of the donor's left atrial appendage. The recipient left atrial appendage is excised, but generally the donor left atrial appendage is left in place. Lower the heart into the pericardium onto a previously placed ice-cold sponge. Continue the anastomosis caudally, along the left side of the left atrium. Run the second arm of Prolene along the dome of the left atrium and then along the interatrial septum. Trim excess cuff tissue, and tie the two arms of suture to complete the left atrial anastomosis (Figs. 5-12 and 5-13).

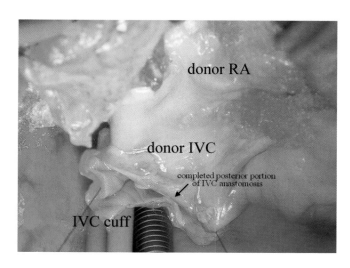

Figure 5-14.

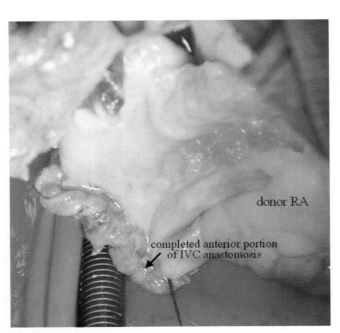

Figure 5-15.

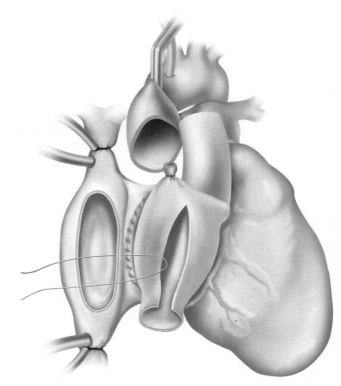

Figure 5-16.

Step 2. IVC anastomosis. For the bicaval method of heart transplantation, anastomose the donor IVC to the recipient IVC in an end-to-end manner with a running 4-0 Prolene suture. Perform the posterior wall of the IVC anastomosis first (Figs. 5-14 and 5-15).

Step 3. Right atrial anastomosis. For the standard method of heart transplantation, after completing the left atrial anastomosis, sew the donor right atrial cuff to the recipient right atrial cuff, beginning along the medial (or septal) edge (Fig. 5-16).

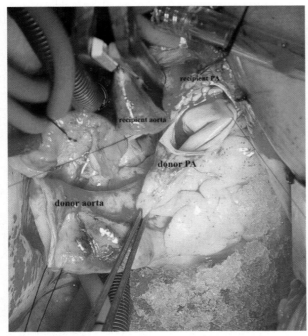

Figure 5-17.

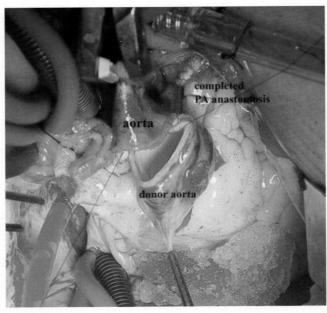

Figure 5-18.

Step 4. Pulmonary artery anastomosis. Anastomose the donor and recipient pulmonary arteries end-to-end with a running 4-0 Prolene suture (Fig. 5-17).

Step 5. Aortic anastomosis. Anastomose the donor and recipient aortas in an end-to-end manner with a running 4-0 Prolene suture (Fig. 5-18).

Step 6. Reperfusion of the heart. After completing the aortic anastomosis, de-air the heart and remove the cross-clamp. This results in reperfusion and ends the graft ischemic period. Before the aortic cross-clamp is removed during the implantation, cold cardioplegia may be administered to reduce graft rewarming. Topical cooling is also used.

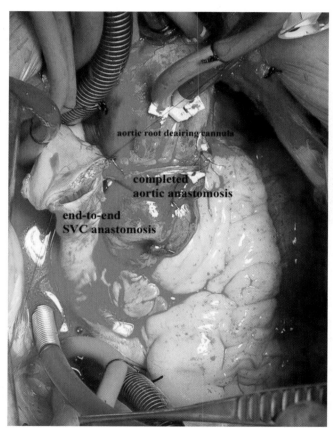

Figure 5-19.

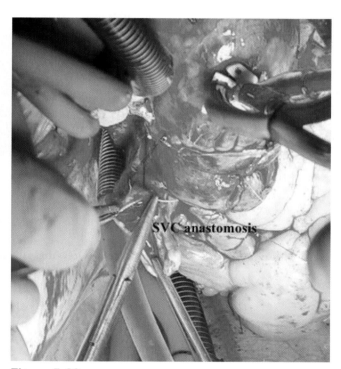

Figure 5-20.

Step 7. Anastomosis of superior vena cava. For the bicaval method of heart transplantation, with the heart reperfused, perform the SVC anastomosis. Sew the donor SVC to the recipient in an end-to-end manner with running 4-0 Prolene. Perform the posterior aspect of the anastomosis first (Figs. 5-19 and 5-20).

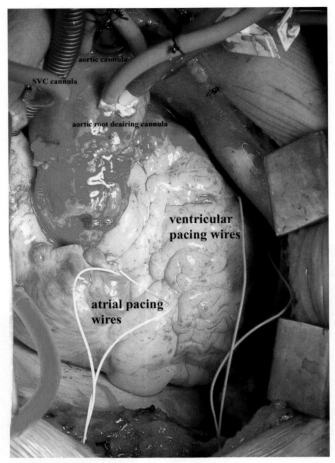

Figure 5-21.

Step 8. Pacing wires. Place atrioventricular epicardial pacing wires and secure them with 6-0 Prolene stitches (Fig. 5-21).

Step 9. Discontinuation of cardiopulmonary bypass. After the anastomoses are inspected for bleeding, the patient is weaned off cardiopulmonary bypass. Usually a reperfusion period of 30 to 60 minutes is helpful before weaning the patient off cardiopulmonary bypass.

Step 10. Removal of cannulas. Remove the IVC cannula and then the SVC cannula. After securing these sites, remove the aortic cannula. Reverse heparin with protamine.

Step 11. Assessment. Assess graft function in the operating room with a pulmonary artery catheter and transesophageal echocardiography. When hemostasis and stable hemodynamics are achieved, place chest tubes in the mediastinum. The pericardium is not closed.

Step 12. Closure. Close the sternotomy with stainless steel wires. Close the overlying fascia and skin with absorbable suture.

Acknowledgment

The authors thank Rick Carver for assisting with intraoperative photography.

Section III

Lung Transplantation

Chapter 6

Lung Transplantation

■ **Matthew G. Hartwig, M.D.**

■ **Shu S. Lin, M.D., Ph.D.**

■ **Sinan A. Simsir, M.D.**

■ **R. Duane Davis, M.D.**

Department of Surgery, Duke University Medical Center, Durham, NC

INTRODUCTION

Two decades separated the first attempt at human lung transplantation by Dr. James Hardy in 1963 at the University of Mississippi and the first successful transplant by Dr. Joel Cooper at the University of Toronto in 1983. However, over the past 20 years, lung transplantation has been shown to be a viable and effective treatment for patients with end-stage lung disease. Progress has been made in surgical techniques, perioperative care, and long-term medical management of this challenging patient population. These refinements in care are reflected by increases in survival over the past 15 years, with 1-year and 3-year survival rates now 76% and 57%, respectively (UNOS 2002 Annual Report).

With such significant improvements in surgical outcomes, the number of potential recipients for lung transplantation has expanded considerably. Although 10,000 lung transplants have been performed since 1988, there are nearly 4,000 persons currently on the lung recipient list, with only 1,000 lung transplants performed in the United States each year (UNOS 2002 Annual Report). This number has remained fairly consistent despite efforts to enlarge the donor pool over the past several years. Of organs commonly transplanted, the lungs are the most sensitive to exogenous damage. Events prior to brain injury, such as smoking, and events associated with brain injury, such as aspiration, mechanical ventilation, or neurogenic pulmonary edema, may compromise the suitability of lungs for transplantation. In addition, to limit ischemia/reperfusion injury, most centers keep total ischemic time of the lungs to less than 6 to 8 hours, restricting the geographic regions of the transplant teams. All of these factors contribute to the imbalance of numbers between lung donors and potential recipients.

In part, subtle yet significant refinements in the surgical procedure over the past 20 years have contributed to improvements in survival. The Toronto Lung Transplant Group initially described a single-lung transplant procedure (Cooper et al, 1987). This is still performed by many centers for nonseptic lung diseases, especially emphysema and pulmonary fibrosis—two of the more common pathologic processes treated with lung transplantation. On the other hand, many centers preferentially perform bilateral sequential lung transplants, regardless of the underlying disease. Internationally, the ratio of single to bilateral lung transplants is approximately equal (ISHLT 2002 Annual Registry). Unless technically not feasible, our group now exclusively performs bilateral sequential single-lung transplants. Cardiopulmonary bypass is avoided through the use of selective lung ventilation whenever possible. This chapter describes the steps in procuring, preparing, and transplanting lungs in a bilateral and sequential fashion. Similar techniques are used when only one lung is being transplanted.

Certain techniques previously described in the literature, such as en-bloc double lung transplants, bronchial artery anastomosis, and omental pedicle flapping, are no longer commonly performed. In the setting of en-bloc transplants, surgeons frequently reported tracheal dehiscence, a devastating complication. Likewise, omental flapping and bronchial artery perfusion, initially used to protect the airway anastomosis, are not common practices at this time. On the other hand, techniques such as using a low-potassium dextran solution for organ preservation, retrograde flushing of the procured organ, and controlling the reperfusion pressure have been shown to decrease injury in animal models and are now routinely performed in human transplantation. Further refinements will certainly be contributed as discoveries are made in basic science and clinical laboratories.

Over the past 40 years lung transplantation has evolved to incorporate a multidisciplinary management group, but patient selection, surgical technique, and perioperative care remain central to advancing the field. Strategies directed toward inducing graft tolerance without generalized immune suppression, advances in infection control, and refinements in surgical technique will improve long-term survival rates. Because of this, the donor pool must be expanded through improvements in preservation techniques, the use of living donors, and the development of the field of xenotransplantation.

SEQUENTIAL BILATERAL LUNG TRANSPLANT RECIPIENT PROCEDURE

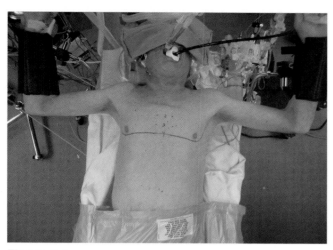

Figure 6-1.

Step 1. Patient positioning and skin incision. With the patient in supine position, both arms are lifted anteriorly and abducted. The forearms are rested on cushioned supports as the arms are flexed slightly at the level of the elbow. An arterial line is placed in the femoral position, and the body below the waist is covered with a warm blanket or heating device. The chest is prepared to the edge of the body laterally where the skin meets the sheet of the operating table. For a male patient (as shown in Fig. 6-1), perform the transsternal bilateral anterior thoracotomy ("clamshell" incision) at the level of the fourth intercostal space.

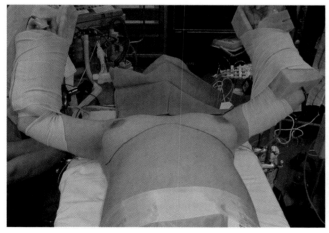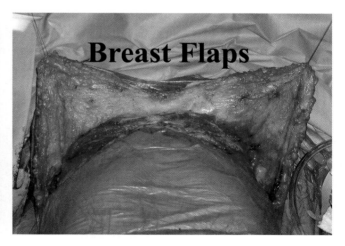

Figure 6-2.

Step 2. Breast flaps for clamshell incision in female patients. For a female patient, make the skin incision at or below the inframammary crease, and open the chest through the fourth intercostal space after a breast flap is developed and retracted superiorly on each side (Fig. 6-2).

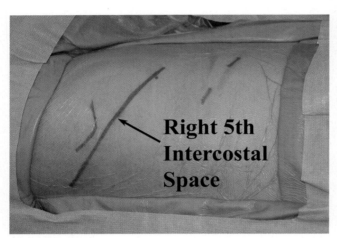

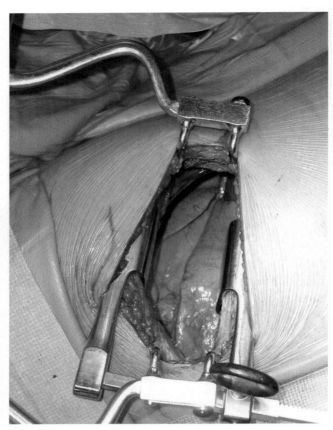

Figure 6-3.

Step 3. Alternative incisions. A muscle-sparing posterolateral thoracotomy through the fifth intercostal space can be used on either side for single-lung transplantation or on both sides as an alternative to the "clamshell" incision described above. Two retractors provide adequate exposure for pneumonectomy and transplant. We primarily use the "clamshell" incision, and the following discussion reflects that bias (Fig. 6-3).

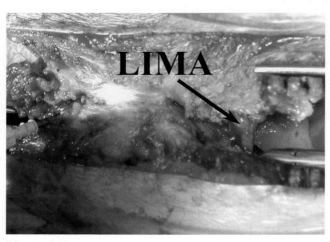

Figure 6-4.

Step 4. Ligation of internal mammary artery. As the "clamshell" thoracotomy is being made, identify the internal mammary artery and vein on each side and ligate them with sutures or metal clips. Shown in Figure 6-4 is the left internal mammary artery (LIMA).

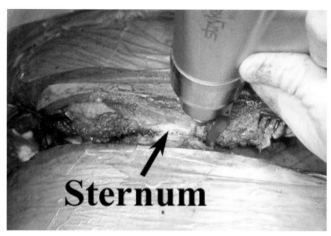

Figure 6-5.

Step 5. Transverse sternotomy to connect the bilateral thoracotomy. Using a sternal saw, divide the midportion of the sternum transversely. Obtain hemostasis of the divided sternum, especially around the posterior table of the sternum (Fig. 6-5).

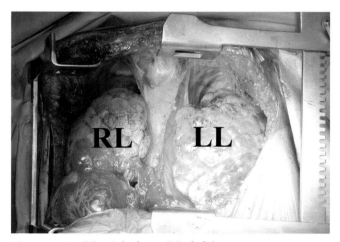

Figure 6-6. RL, right lung; LL, left lung.

Step 6. Initial exposure of the "clamshell" incision. As chest wall retractors are placed on each side, you will be able to appreciate the overall exposure to both diseased lungs. The pericardium should remain intact at this point but may be opened if the use of cardiopulmonary bypass is anticipated (see next step) (Fig. 6-6).

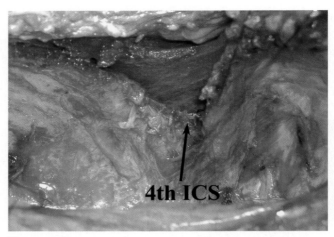

Figure 6-7.

Step 7. Release of intercostal muscles. To maximize the overall exposure with this incision, divide the bilateral intercostal muscles in the fourth intercostal space (ICS). The overlying muscles (e.g., latissimus dorsi and serratus anterior) are relatively spared laterally (Fig. 6-7).

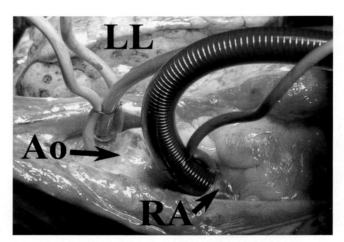

Figure 6-8. LL, left lung; Ao, aorta; RA, right atrium.

Step 8. Placement of arterial and venous cannulas for cardiopulmonary bypass. This step can be performed at this point when planned ahead or at any point in the operation as needed. Intravenous heparin is administered before cannulation, or before mobilization and division of hilar structures (see below) if cardiopulmonary bypass is not used (Fig. 6-8).

RIGHT LUNG TRANSPLANTATION

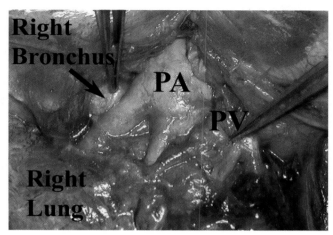

Figure 6-9.

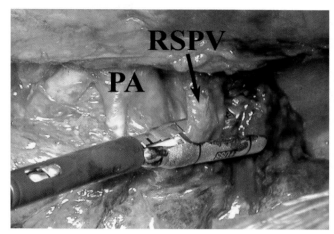

Figure 6-10.

Step 1. Exposure of the right hilum. As you selectively deflate the right lung, the hilum is exposed and you can immediately identify the superior pulmonary vein (PV) and most of the pulmonary artery (PA). Take down pleural adhesions. Divide the mediastinal pleura to mobilize the hilar structures (Fig. 6-9).

Step 2. Mobilization and division of right superior pulmonary vein (RSPV). Mobilize the superior pulmonary vein, the most accessible vascular structure in the hilum, and divide it using an Endo-GIA stapler. The inferior pulmonary vein can be mobilized and divided later, as the exposure of this structure improves after the right pulmonary artery (PA) is divided and mobilized (Fig. 6-10).

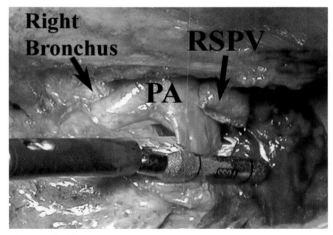

Figure 6-11.

Step 3. Mobilization and division of right pulmonary artery. Carefully mobilize the branches of the right pulmonary artery. Figure 6-11 shows the division of the ongoing pulmonary artery using an Endo-GIA stapler. This step facilitates mobilization of the anterior trunk of the right pulmonary artery.

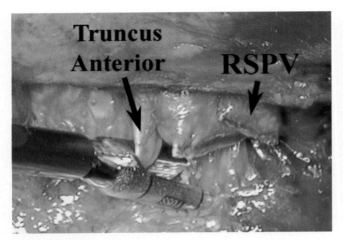

Truncus Anterior   RSPV

Figure 6-12.

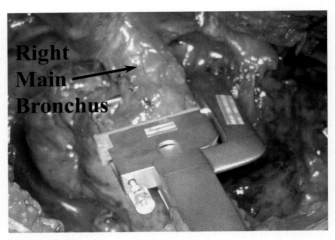

Right Main Bronchus

Figure 6-13.

Step 4. Division of the anterior trunk of the right pulmonary artery. Using an Endo-GIA stapler, divide the truncus anterior, which separates into the apical and anterior branches of the right pulmonary artery. After dividing the arterial structures, divide the inferior pulmonary ligament, and mobilize the inferior pulmonary vein and divide it with an Endo-GIA stapler (Fig. 6-12).

Step 5. Mobilization and division of the right bronchus. When mobilized sufficiently, the right mainstem bronchus can be divided with the stapler at the most distal segment just before the takeoff of the right upper lobe bronchus (Fig. 6-13).

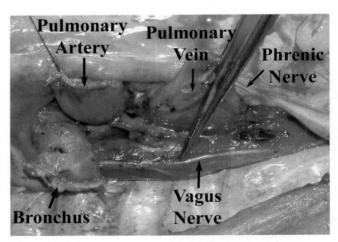

Pulmonary Artery   Pulmonary Vein   Phrenic Nerve

Bronchus   Vagus Nerve

Figure 6-14.

Step 6. Removal of recipient native right lung and exposure of the divided bronchovascular structure. Divide the remaining pleural adhesions. When you encounter adhesions medially, take care not to injure the phrenic nerve, which lies anterior to the hilar structures that were divided. After the native right lung is removed, the exposure of the divided bronchovascular structures and their surrounding tissue is the greatest, and it is at this time that selective hemostasis is best achieved (Fig. 6-14).

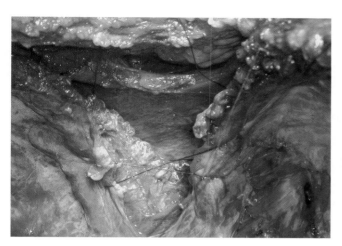

Figure 6-15.

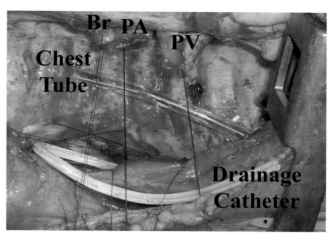

Figure 6-16. Br, bronchus; PA, pulmonary artery; PV, pulmonary vein.

Step 7. Placement of pericostal sutures laterally. Place two sets of figure-of-eight #1 Maxon pericostal sutures in the intercostal release incisions in preparation for closure of the chest because of the excellent exposure obtained while the lung is out of the pleural cavity (Fig. 6-15).

Step 8. Placement of posterior chest tube and axillary drainage tube. Insert a large-bore chest tube through a separate skin incision inferior to the "clamshell" incision and position it posteriorly in the pleural cavity. A smaller-caliber suction catheter placed into this chest tube and connected to a suction device then facilitates the drainage of blood and fluid throughout the case. A flexible drainage tube can also be placed at this time in the axillary space, between the rib cage and the latissimus muscle; in female patients, the tip of this catheter can later be guided into the submammary space near the end of the operation (Fig. 6-16).

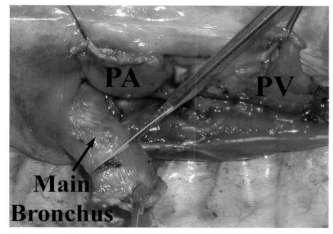

Figure 6-17.

Step 9. Preparation of the recipient right mainstem bronchus. Cut the right mainstem bronchus with a #10 blade just proximal to the takeoff of the right upper lobe bronchus (Fig. 6-17).

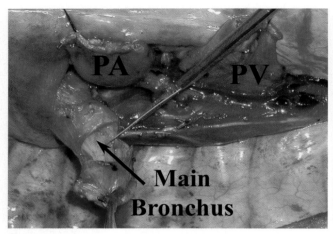

Figure 6-18.

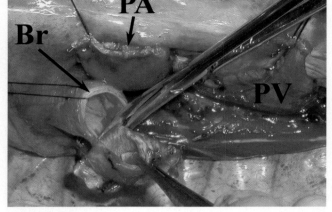

Figure 6-19.

Step 10. Preparation of the recipient right mainstem bronchus (2). As more of the bronchial wall is cut with a #10 blade, use a suction device to remove any mucus or secretion noted within the lumen (Fig. 6-18).

Step 11. Preparation of the recipient right mainstem bronchus (3). After dividing the cartilaginous portion of the bronchus with a blade, place a retraction stitch anteriorly to secure control of the bronchus. Then divide the remainder of the bronchial wall (posterior, membranous portion) with sharp scissors (Fig. 6-19).

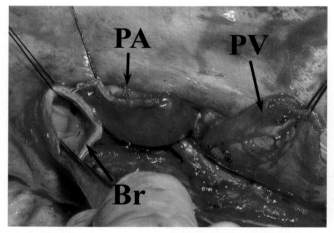

Figure 6-20.

Step 12. The recipient right mainstem bronchus, prepared. The recipient bronchus is now ready for anastomosis. Aspirate any secretions within the lumen. Use antibiotic solution to irrigate the lumen of the right mainstem bronchus. The endotracheal tube intubating the left mainstem bronchus is clearly visible from the open lumen of the distal right mainstem bronchus (Fig. 6-20).

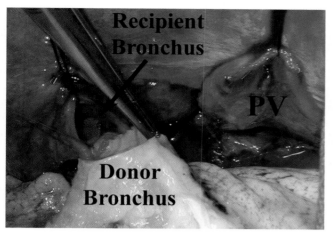

Figure 6-21.

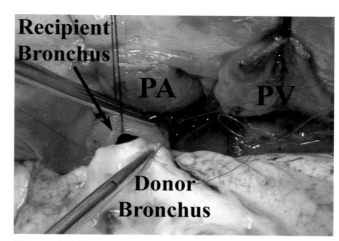

Figure 6-22.

Step 13. Right bronchial anastomosis—posterior row. Place cold laparotomy sponges posteriorly in the pleural cavity, and orthotopically position the donor right lung in the pleural cavity. Align the recipient bronchus and donor bronchus, and perform the bronchial anastomosis with a running 4-0 PDS suture. As shown in Figure 6-21, the posterior, membranous portion of the bronchial anastomosis is performed first, starting from one corner of the membranocartilaginous junction.

Step 14. Right bronchial anastomosis—anterior row. Anastomose the anterior, cartilaginous portion of the bronchus. Placement of a transition stitch in the opposing corner creates an intussusception, usually of the donor bronchus into the recipient bronchus. Thus, the orientation of the anatomy is preserved with membranous-to-membranous and cartilaginous-to-cartilaginous apposition (Fig. 6-22).

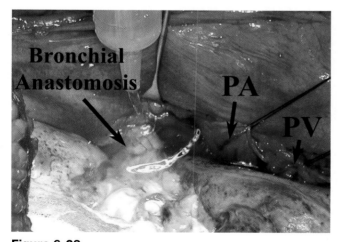

Figure 6-23.

Step 15. Testing of the bronchial anastomosis. Evaluate the right bronchial anastomosis for an obvious air leak under water while the anesthesiologist manually inflates the right lung with room air (Fig. 6-23).

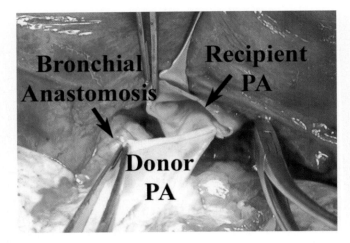

Figure 6-24.

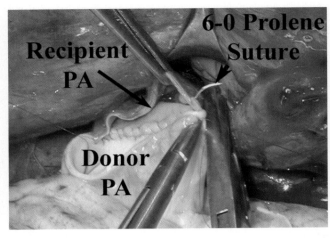

Figure 6-25.

Step 16. Preparation of right pulmonary artery anastomosis. After completing the bronchial anastomosis, occlude the stapled recipient right pulmonary artery proximally with a Satinsky vascular clamp, and trim away the staple line. Similarly, trim the donor pulmonary artery to an appropriate length. Take care not to leave the donor or recipient pulmonary artery too long as to cause kinking after the anastomosis is made. Then align the recipient pulmonary artery and the donor pulmonary artery in preparation for the anastomosis, which is begun in one corner with running 6-0 Prolene (Fig. 6-24).

Step 17. Right pulmonary artery anastomosis, posterior row. Figure 6-25 shows a magnified view of the posterior row. Continue the running 6-0 Prolene on the anterior row.

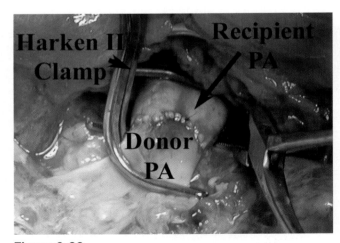

Figure 6-26.

Step 18. Completed right pulmonary artery anastomosis. Test the newly created right pulmonary artery anastomosis by placing a second vascular clamp (e.g., Harken II) distal to the anastomosis on the donor pulmonary artery and removing the previously placed Satinsky clamp on the recipient pulmonary artery (Fig. 6-26).

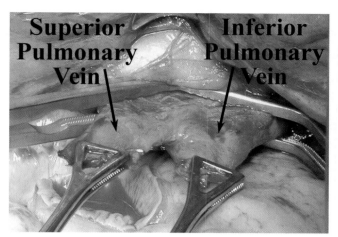

Figure 6-27.

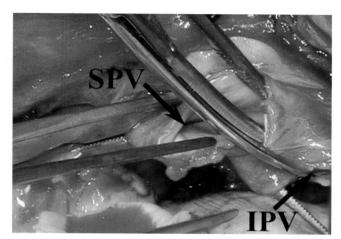

Figure 6-28.

Step 19. Preparation of recipient left atrial cuff for pulmonary venous anastomosis on the right side. As you retract the stapled superior and inferior right pulmonary vein stumps laterally with Pennington clamps, place a large Satinsky vascular clamp toward the body of the left atrium. Trim each of the staple lines (Fig. 6-27).

Step 20. Preparation of recipient left atrial cuff for pulmonary venous anastomosis on the right side (2). Connect the orifices of the superior pulmonary vein (SPV) and inferior pulmonary vein (IPV) with sharp scissors, creating a large recipient left atrial cuff on the right side (Fig. 6-28).

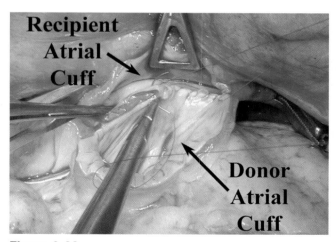

Figure 6-29.

Step 21. Connection of the pulmonary venous system. Using a running 5-0 Prolene suture, anastomose the left atrial cuff of the donor right lung to the common opening created between the recipient's right superior and inferior pulmonary veins (recipient left atrial cuff). Intimal apposition is achieved without including much of the excess tissue beyond the muscular layer. Shown in Figure 6-29 is the start of the posterior row anastomosis as the anterior lip of the recipient left atrial cuff is retracted up with a Pennington clamp.

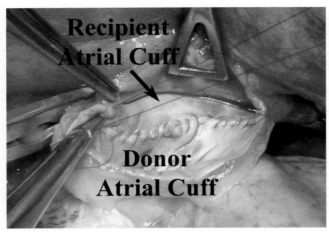

Figure 6-30.

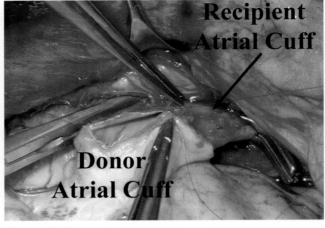

Figure 6-31.

Step 22. Connection of the pulmonary venous system (2). Complete the posterior row of the pulmonary venous anastomosis (Fig. 6-30).

Step 23. Connection of the pulmonary venous system (3). Continue the same running 5-0 Prolene suture on the anterior row. An intravenous bolus of methylprednisolone (500 mg) and mannitol (25 g) are given immediately before this step is completed (Fig. 6-31).

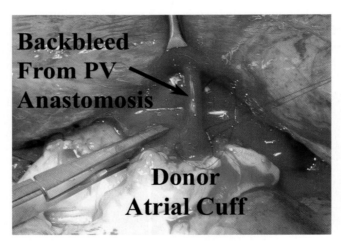

Figure 6-32.

Step 24. De-airing of the pulmonary vascular bed and reperfusion of the transplanted lung. With the last few throws of the 5-0 Prolene suture left loose anteriorly, partially release the vascular clamp on the pulmonary artery to allow blood to flow into the newly implanted right lung through the right pulmonary artery anastomosis in order to remove air from within the pulmonary vasculature. Immediately before tying down the 5-0 Prolene suture, release the Satinsky clamp on the recipient left atrium to force out any residual air. Controlled, low-pressure perfusion of the lung is achieved by gradually releasing the pulmonary artery clamp over 10 to 15 minutes. Ventilation with room air is initiated by hand and then continued with mechanical ventilation. The pressure-control mode of ventilation is preferred with 5 to 8 cm of positive end-expiratory pressure, distending pressure of 16 to 22 cm, and minimal FiO_2—preferably less than 30% (Fig. 6-32).

LEFT LUNG TRANSPLANTATION

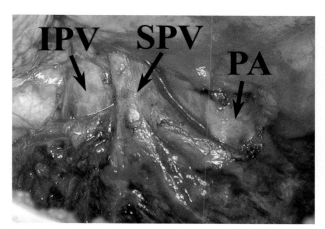

Figure 6-33.

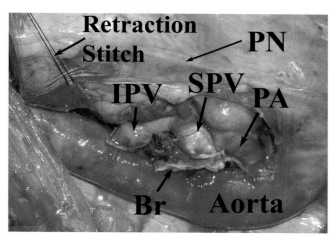

Figure 6-34.

Step 1. Exposure of the left hilum. As the left lung is selectively deflated, the hilum is exposed. Identify the superior pulmonary vein (SPV), inferior pulmonary vein (IPV), and left main pulmonary artery (PA). Again, carefully take down pleural and mediastinal adhesions, if present (Fig. 6-33).

Step 2. Preparation of left hilar structures. After opening the pleura and the pericardium medially on the left side, individually staple each of the hilar bronchovascular structures, including the superior pulmonary vein (SPV), inferior pulmonary vein (IPV), left pulmonary artery (PA), and left main bronchus (Br), and divide them in a manner similar to the right side. Place a heavy silk retraction stitch inferiorly on the pericardium, posterior to the phrenic nerve (PN) and anterior to the inferior pulmonary vein (Fig. 6-34).

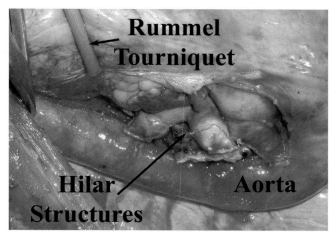

Figure 6-35.

Step 3. Rummel tourniquet on the retraction stitch. A heavy-duty Rummel tourniquet (e.g., fashioned from a red Robinson catheter) is used to reinforce the retraction stitch so that the heart can be safely retracted upward and to the right to improve exposure during further dissection of the hilar structures and implantation of the donor lung (Fig. 6-35).

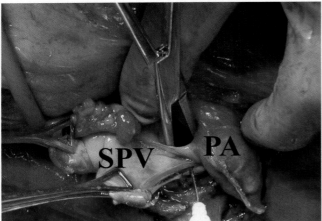

Figure 6-36.

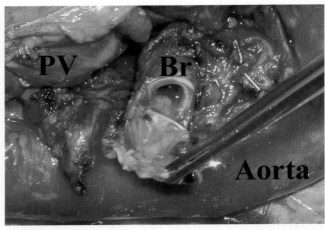

Figure 6-37.

Step 4. Dissection of the hilar structures. Divide the tissue connecting the left pulmonary artery and the left superior pulmonary vein and carefully obtain hemostasis (Fig. 6-36).

Step 5. Preparation of the recipient left mainstem bronchus. After placing the posterior chest tubes and the axillary drainage tube as described for the right side, prepare the recipient left mainstem bronchus (Br) by dividing it with a fresh #10 blade just proximal to the staple line (Fig. 6-37).

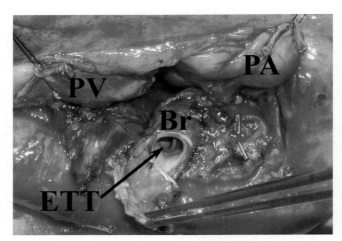

Figure 6-38.

Step 6. Preparation of the recipient left mainstem bronchus (2). After any mucus or secretions are removed from the lumen of the bronchus with a suction device, the tip of the endotracheal tube (ETT) is visible. Similar to the right side, place a retraction stitch anteriorly to assist in the exposure of the left bronchus (Fig. 6-38).

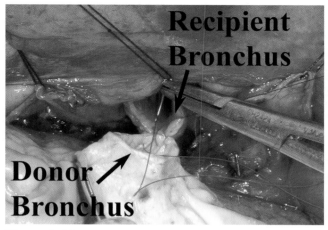

Figure 6-39.

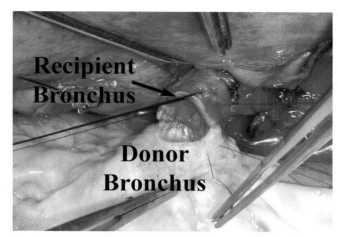

Figure 6-40.

Step 7. Left bronchial anastomosis, posterior row. Perform the left bronchial anastomosis just as you did on the right side. Place cold laparotomy sponges posteriorly in the pleural cavity, and position the donor left lung orthotopically in the pleural cavity. Align the recipient bronchus and donor bronchus, and perform the bronchial anastomosis with a running 4-0 PDS suture. Again, as shown in Figure 6-39, perform the posterior, membranous portion of the bronchial anastomosis first, starting from one corner of the membranocartilaginous junction.

Step 8. Left bronchial anastomosis, anterior row. Continue the anterior row of the left bronchial anastomosis as described for the right side (Fig. 6-40).

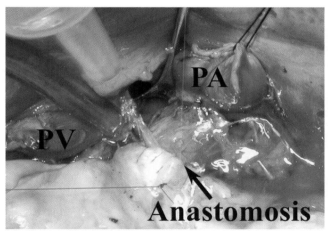

Figure 6-41.

Step 9. Testing of bronchial anastomosis. Check the left bronchial anastomosis for an obvious air leak under water while the anesthesiologist manually inflates the left lung (Fig. 6-41).

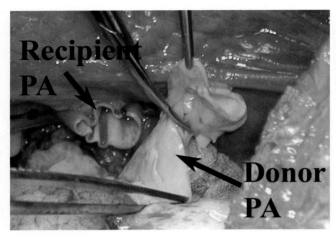

Figure 6-42.

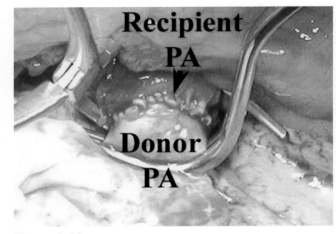

Figure 6-43.

Step 10. Preparation of left pulmonary artery anastomosis. After completing the bronchial anastomosis, prepare the recipient and donor left pulmonary arteries just as described for the right side. As shown in Figure 6-42, the stapled recipient left pulmonary artery has already been occluded proximally with a Satinsky vascular clamp and the staple line trimmed away. Trim the donor left pulmonary artery to an appropriate length so as to avoid kinking of the vessel after the anastomosis. Then align the recipient pulmonary artery and the donor pulmonary artery in preparation for the anastomosis, which is performed with running 6-0 Prolene.

Step 11. Completed left pulmonary artery anastomosis. Test the newly created left pulmonary anastomosis by placing a second vascular clamp (e.g., Harken II) distal to the anastomosis on the donor pulmonary artery and removing the previously placed Satinsky clamp on the recipient pulmonary artery (Fig. 6-43).

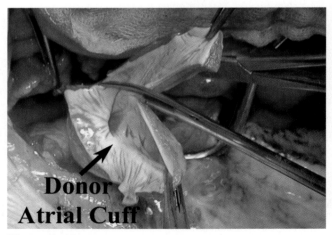

Figure 6-44.

Step 12. Preparation of donor atrial cuff for pulmonary venous anastomosis on the left side. Identify the superior and inferior pulmonary veins within the atrial cuff of the donor left lung. Trim the atrial cuff to an appropriate size in preparation for pulmonary venous anastomosis. (Fig. 6-44).

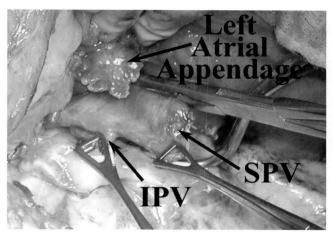

Figure 6-45.

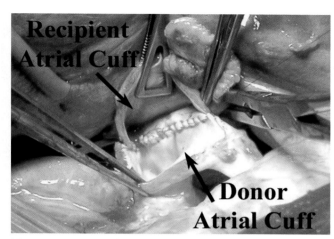

Figure 6-46.

Step 13. Preparation of recipient left atrial cuff for pulmonary venous anastomosis on the left side. As the stapled superior pulmonary vein (SPV) and inferior pulmonary vein (IPV) stumps are retracted laterally with Pennington clamps, place a large Satinsky vascular clamp toward the body of the left atrium. Trim each of the staple lines. Then connect the orifices of the superior and inferior pulmonary veins with sharp scissors, creating a large recipient left atrial cuff (Fig. 6-45).

Step 14. Connection of the pulmonary venous system. Using a running 5-0 Prolene suture, anastomose the atrial cuff of the donor left lung to the common opening created between the recipient's left superior and inferior pulmonary veins (i.e., recipient left atrial cuff). Intimal apposition is achieved without including excess tissue beyond the muscular layer. Figure 6-46 shows the completion of the posterior row anastomosis as the anterior lip of the recipient left atrial cuff is retracted anteriorly with a Pennington clamp.

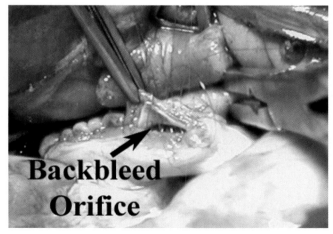

Figure 6-47.

Step 15. Connection of the pulmonary venous system (2). The anterior row of the pulmonary venous anastomosis is nearly completed. As shown in Figure 6-47, leave the running 5-0 Prolene suture loose at the end for back-bleeding in order to de-air the pulmonary vascular bed. An intravenous bolus of methylprednisolone (500 mg) and mannitol (25 g) are given immediately before completion of this step.

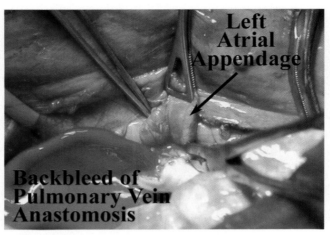

Figure 6-48.

Step 16. De-airing of the pulmonary vascular bed and reperfusion of the transplanted lung. Partially release the vascular clamp on the pulmonary artery to allow blood to flow into the transplanted left lung through the pulmonary artery anastomosis in order to remove air from within the pulmonary vasculature. Immediately before tying down the suture, release the Satinsky clamp on the recipient left atrium to force any residual air out of the left atrium. As previously described, the pulmonary artery clamp is gradually released over a period of 10 to 15 minutes to achieve controlled reperfusion of the transplanted left lung (Fig. 6-48).

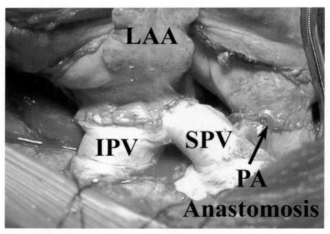

Figure 6-49.

Step 17. Completed pulmonary venous connection on the left side. The recipient left atrial appendage (LAA) is retracted anteriorly as the completed pulmonary venous anastomosis is shown for the left lung (Fig. 6-49). The pulmonary artery clamp is now completely released, thereby allowing full flow through the pulmonary artery anastomosis. Ventilation with room air is initiated by hand, followed by mechanical ventilation. The pressure-control mode of ventilation is preferred, with a distending pressure of 16 to 22 cm, positive end-expiratory pressure of 5 to 8 cm, and minimal FiO_2, optimally less than 30%.

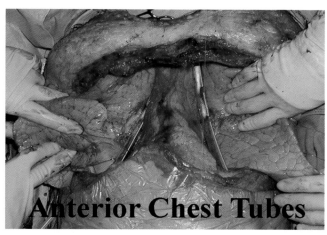

Figure 6-50.

Step 18. Placement of anterior chest tubes. Place 32- or 36-Fr drainage tubes anteriorly, just underneath the medial surface of the upper lobes, and bring them out through separate stab incisions inferiorly (Fig. 6-50).

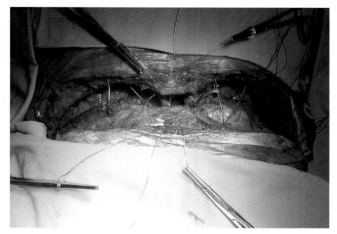

Figure 6-51.

Step 19. Closing wires and sutures. Approximate the anterior aspect of the "clamshell" opening with three sets of #5 wires—one simple set in the midline of the sternum and one set of figure-of-eight on each side of the midline. Reapprox-imate the remainder of the "clamshell" opening with a series of #1 Maxon sutures in figure-of-eight fashion. As described earlier, the Maxon sutures in the most lat-eral aspect of the opening were placed while the native lungs were either deflated or removed. If not already done, place a Blake drain into each of the axillary spaces. Approximate the pectoral fascial layer, the subcutaneous layer, the subdermal layer, and the skin (Fig. 6-51).

REFERENCES

1. Cooper JD, Pearson FG, Patterson GA, et al. Technique of successful lung transplantation in humans. *J Thorac Cardiovasc Surg* 1987;93:173–181.
2. URREA; UNOS. *2002 Annual Report of the U.S. Organ Procurement and Transplantation Network and the Scientific Registry of Transplant Recipients: Transplant Data 1992–2001* [Internet]. Rockville, MD: HHS/HRSA/OSP/DOT; 2003 [modified Feb. 18, 2003; cited Oct. 20, 2003].
3. Hertz MI, Taylor DO, Trulock EP, et al. The Registry of the International Society for Heart and Lung Transplantation: 19th official report, 2002. *J Heart Lung Transplant* 2002;21:950–970.

Chapter 7
Heart-Lung Transplantation

■ **Matthew G. Hartwig, M.D.**

Department of Surgery, Duke University Medical
Center, Durham, NC

■ **Steven S. L. Tsui, M.D., F.R.C.S.**

Papworth Hospital, Cambridge, United Kingdom

INTRODUCTION

Heart-lung transplantation is performed under general anesthesia with the recipient in the supine position. A radial artery line, internal jugular venous sheath, and urinary catheter are placed and the patient is intubated with a single-lumen endotracheal tube. The venous sheath can be used to facilitate placement of the pulmonary artery (PA) catheter at the end of the operation, if one is desired. The PA catheter can be advanced safely following completion of the superior vena cava (SVC) anastomosis. Prophylactic antibiotics are given and a test dose of aprotinin (50,000 U or 5 mL) is administered by slow intravenous injection to exclude allergy. This test dose is given sufficiently early so that cardiopulmonary bypass could be rapidly initiated if needed. If tolerated, the recipient is given 2 million units (200 mL) of aprotinin intravenously as a loading dose over 20 minutes, and a further 2 million units of aprotinin is added to the priming fluid of the bypass circuit. The maintenance dose of aprotinin is 0.5 million units per hour (50 mL/hr) throughout the procedure and until the recipient is stable in the intensive care unit.

Heart-lung transplantation is most commonly performed through a median sternotomy incision. This approach allows excellent exposure of all the mediastinal structures as well as access to the hilum of both lungs. This incision may be extended above the sternal notch if the innominate vein is to be cannulated for cardiopulmonary bypass. An alternative approach is via the "clamshell" incision, or bilateral thoracosternotomy. This can be used when extensive pleural adhesions are anticipated, as this incision provides superior surgical access to the lateral and posterior aspects of the pleural spaces. Pleural adhesions can be highly vascular and are best divided with electrocautery before the patient is systemically heparinized. After establishing hemostasis of the pleural adhesions, heparin is given intravenously for systemic anticoagulation (300 U/kg to achieve an activated clotting time of more than 700 seconds with the Hemochron 801 or more than 400 seconds with the ACT II). The anterior pericardium is now opened with an inverted-T incision and two strong stay sutures are placed on each side of the pericardial edge. Traction on these sutures will facilitate subsequent exposure of the hilar structures.

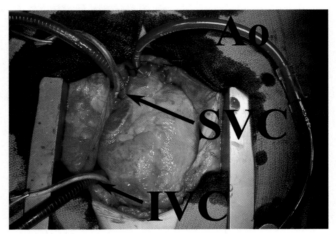

Figure 7-1.

Step 1. Cannulation. Cardiopulmonary bypass (CPB) is instituted. Separate the ascending aorta from the pulmonary trunk. Dissect free both venae cavae and encircle them with nylon tapes. Perform standard high ascending aortic cannulation with a 24-gauge aortic cannula (Ao) for arterial return. Cannulate the superior vena cava (SVC) with a 28-gauge right-angled cannula for head and neck venous drainage. Separately cannulate the inferior vena cava (IVC) with a 30-gauge straight cannula. If the recipient's heart is to be used as a domino donor heart, place the IVC cannula as far lateral and inferior as possible in order to leave sufficient margins of atrial tissue on the domino donor heart and for subsequent anastomosis of the IVC to the donor heart-lung bloc. CPB is commenced, the patient is cooled to 30°C, and ventilation is discontinued (Fig. 7-1).

An alternative to SVC cannulation for head and neck drainage is direct cannulation of the innominate vein. Separating the two lobes of the overlying thymic remnant with electrocautery exposes the vein. Place a 5-0 polypropylene purse-string suture in the center of the innominate vein. This purse-string suture is diamond-shaped and should lie along the length of the vein, approximately 8 mm wide and 15 mm long. Use tissue forceps to steady the vein on either side of the purse-string suture and make a 12-mm incision in the vein with a #11 scalpel blade in the center of the purse-string. A 20- or 22-gauge straight venous cannula can be inserted vertically into the vein to a depth of 1 cm, and the 5-0 purse-string suture is tightened with a snare. This allows drainage of the innominate vein from both sides of the cannula. Secure this venous cannula against the skin edge to prevent it from being dislodged during the rest of the procedure (not pictured).

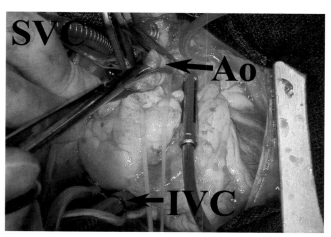

Figure 7-2.

Step 2. Division of ascending aorta. One of the most important aspects of heart-lung transplantation is to avoid injury to the nerves travelling through the mediastinum. Preservation of the phrenic nerves, the vagus nerves, and the left recurrent laryngeal nerve in the recipient can be achieved by careful dissection and excision of the recipient heart and lungs. First, apply a cross-clamp to the distal ascending aorta (Ao). If the recipient's heart is used for domino donation, cardioplegia is delivered into the aortic root for myocardial preservation and ice slurry is added to the pericardium for topical cooling. Once the heart is arrested, the SVC is clamped cranial to the right atrium, the nylon tape is tightened around the IVC, and the recipient's heart can be excised. Figure 7-2 shows the ascending aorta being divided approximately 1 cm above the sino-tubular junction.

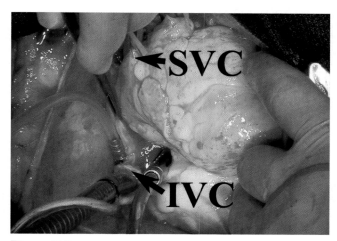

Figure 7-3.

Step 3. Division of SVC and IVC. Divide the SVC close to the atrial-caval junction so as to maximize the length of the recipient SVC. For a domino heart, the SVC is divided 1 cm cranial to the atrial-caval junction to avoid damaging the sinoatrial node. After dividing the SVC, turn your attention to the IVC. In Figure 7-3, the assistant retracts the heart to the left for proper exposure of the IVC. Make the incision in the IVC so as to leave a 1-cm cuff of tissue around the IVC cannula to facilitate subsequent implantation. The rest of the cardiectomy is similar to that of a cadaveric donor heart, with division of the individual pulmonary veins, the distal pulmonary trunk, and the posterior pericardial reflections behind the roof of the left atrium.

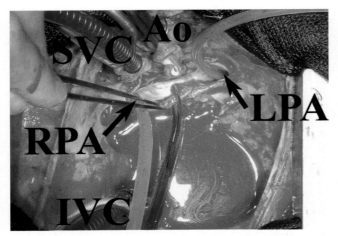

Figure 7-4. LPA, left pulmonary artery; RPA, right pulmonary artery; SVC, superior vena cava; IVC, inferior vena cava.

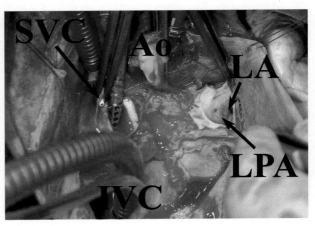

Figure 7-5.

Step 4. Bisection of pulmonary trunk. Following recipient cardiectomy, the next step is to bisect the pulmonary trunk at its bifurcation into the right and left pulmonary arteries (Fig. 7-4).

Step 5. Locating the left recurrent laryngeal nerve. Since the left recurrent laryngeal nerve passes under the aortic arch adjacent to the ligamentum arteriosum, take special care in this area to avoid injuring it. A dimple on the intimal surface of the left pulmonary artery (LPA) marks the site of the ligamentum arteriosum (LA) (Fig. 7-5).

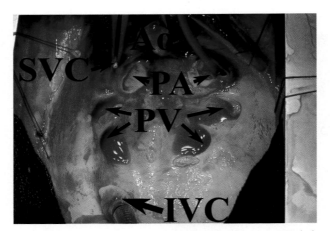

Figure 7-6. PA, left and right pulmonary artery; PV, left inferior and superior and right inferior and superior pulmonary veins.

Step 6. Protecting the left recurrent laryngeal nerve. Leave a patch of PA attached to the ligamentum arteriosum by making a circular incision in the roof of the left PA, keeping 5 to 8 mm away from the dimple of the ligamentum arteriosum. Leaving this 1-cm disc of PA on the underside of the aortic arch avoids injury to the left recurrent laryngeal nerve. Avoid using electrocautery, and control bleeding points with Ligaclips. Use scissors to dissect the rest of the left and right PAs free laterally toward the lungs. Figure 7-6 shows the pericardial sac with its vascular structures nearly ready for subsequent anastomosis.

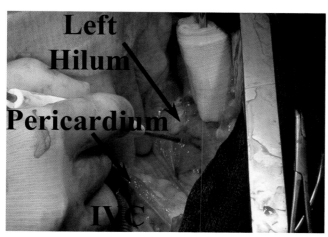

Figure 7-7.

Step 7. Exposing the hilum of the left lung. Dissect the anterior hilum of the lung. Widely open the pleural reflection along the cut edge of the pericardium, and bring the left-sided pericardial stay sutures over to the right side of the chest. To expose the hilum of the left lung, the surgeon retracts the pericardium toward the right and the assistant provides countertraction on the upper lobe of the lung (Fig. 7-7).

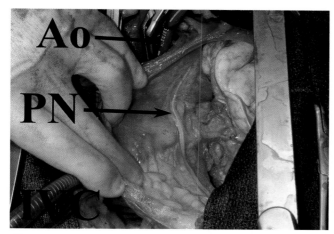

Figure 7-8.

Step 8. Identification of left phrenic nerve (PN). The left lung is initially mobilized by dividing the pulmonary ligament with electrocautery. Then incise the anterior pleural reflection overlying the left PA and veins. The left phrenic nerve can be clearly seen lying on the lateral surface of the pericardium en route to the diaphragm. This is usually a good distance anterior to the left hilum (Fig. 7-8).

Step 9. Creation of pericardial windows. Incise the pericardium adjacent to the pulmonary vessels. As the pericardial sac is cut open, the stumps of the pulmonary veins together with the stump of the left PA can be delivered into the pleural cavity. Traction on these vessels will allow extension of the incision in the pericardium to encircle the pulmonary veins. This creates a small aperture in the left lateral aspect of the posterior pericardial sac. Extending the incision inferiorly toward the diaphragm enlarges the pericardial window and facilitates subsequent passage of the left donor lung through this aperture.

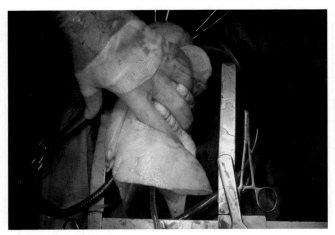

Figure 7-9.

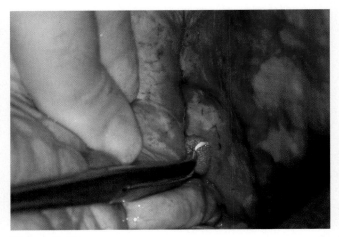

Figure 7-10.

Step 10. Exposure of posterior hilar structures. Dissect the posterior lung hilum. Bring the left lung out of the wound and retract it toward the right of midline to expose the posterior aspect of the left hilum (Fig. 7-9).

Step 11. Protecting the left vagus nerve. The vagus nerves pass inferiorly in the posterior mediastinum behind the left main bronchi. Even though it may not be easily identifiable at this stage, the left vagus nerve is often stretched across the posterior surface of the left main bronchus. To avoid injury to this nerve, the pleural reflections overlying the left main bronchus must be incised close to the lung substance. Then sweep the pleura away from the surface of the bronchus toward the mediastinum using a dental swab mounted on a Roberts clamp (Fig. 7-10).

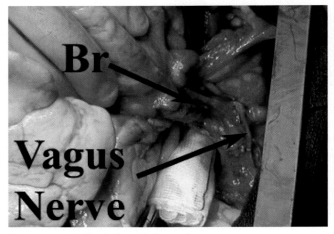

Figure 7-11. Br, left main bronchus.

Step 12. Ligation and division of bronchial artery. Branches of the bronchial artery are ligated before they are divided. Once this has been completed, the intact left vagus nerve is often seen lying close to the cut edge of the pleural reflection on the anterior surface of the exposed esophagus (Fig. 7-11).

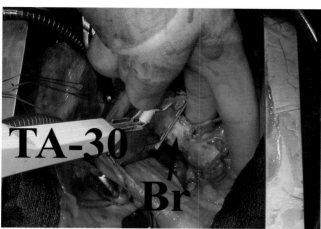

Figure 7-12.

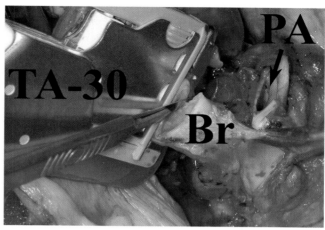

Figure 7-13.

Step 13. Dissecting the left main bronchus. Return the left lung to the pleural cavity. Divide the remaining soft tissue and lymph nodes on its anterior surface with electrocautery to skeletonize the left main bronchus. Seal the bronchus with a TA-30 stapling device (Fig. 7-12).

Step 14. Excision of left lung. Dividing the bronchus distal to the staples allows excision of the lung without contamination of the operative field by the bronchial stump (Fig. 7-13).

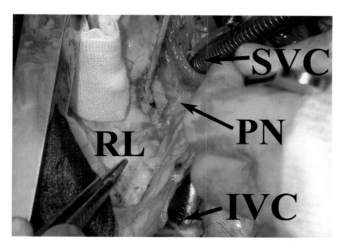

Figure 7-14.

Step 15. Excision of right lung. Dissect the right lung free (RL) and excise it in a similar manner by repeating the steps above. The right phrenic nerve (PN) tends to lie much closer to the right lung hilum, so take special care to avoid injuring it. In Figure 7-14, the blue electrocautery device is shown dividing along the pleural reflection.

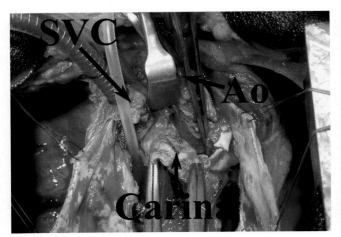

Figure 7-15.

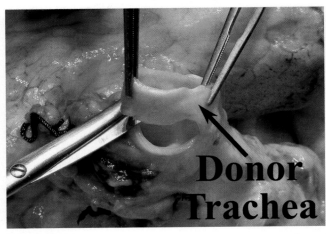

Figure 7-16.

Step 16. Preparation of trachea. Once both recipient lungs have been excised, the two previously stapled bronchial stumps become visible through the central defect in the posterior pericardium. The anesthesiologist should clear the recipient trachea of collected secretions with a suction catheter. Introducing 30 mL of 10% aqueous Betadine solution directly into the endotracheal tube washes out the airway. Apply tissue clamps to each of the two bronchial stumps, and bring the tracheal carina into the operating field by downward traction on the bronchial stumps. Swivelling the aortic cross-clamp counterclockwise widens the space between the SVC and the ascending aorta and enhances access to the tracheal carina. Bulky soft tissue overlying the trachea can also be retracted gently upward (Fig. 7-15).

Step 17. Exposing the carina. A sleeve of fibrofatty tissue and carinal lymph nodes envelops the distal trachea and the tracheal carina. Use electrocautery to make a transverse incision into this pericarinal tissue envelope. This incision should be made as low as possible so as not to disturb the blood supply of the distal trachea. To excise the tracheal carina and the bronchial stumps, they need to be skeletonized by blunt dissection using a dental swab. The posterior surface of the carina is exposed by anterior traction on the bronchial stumps. Both vagus nerves are at further risk of injury during this maneuver as they become tented forward by the traction on the bronchi. Avoid the use of electrocautery for this dissection, and keep the plane of blunt dissection right on the surface of the airways. At this stage, dissection of the mediastinum is almost complete. Before continuing any further, carry out meticulous hemostasis of all the posterior mediastinal structures, because these areas will be rendered inaccessible once the donor organs have been inserted.

Step 18. Preparing donor airways for implantation. After inspection and orientation of the donor heart-lung bloc, transect the donor trachea 2 cm above the carina. Leave the pericarinal fibrofatty envelope on the donor carina undisturbed to preserve the blood supply to the donor airways. Aspirate secretions from the donor airways and send them for microbiologic examination. Gently wash out each donor bronchus with 20 mL normal saline to remove retained secretions. Trim the donor trachea to its final length for implantation with scalpel and scissors. This should be just one cartilage ring above the carina (Fig. 7-16).

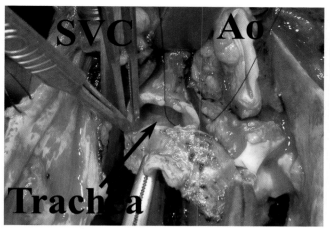

Figure 7-17.

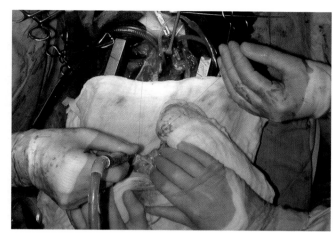

Figure 7-18.

Step 19. Transection of recipient trachea. Once the donor heart-lung bloc has been prepared, open the recipient trachea just above the carina by a transverse incision using a no. 11 scalpel blade. Avoid the use of electrocautery in this area, and leave the peritracheal soft tissue envelope undisturbed to preserve the blood supply to the recipient side of the tracheal anastomosis. Carry the tracheal incision around the anterior two-thirds of the trachea (Fig. 7-17).

Step 20. Preparation for airway anastomosis. At this stage, traction on the tracheal stump is maintained through the membranous part of the trachea to prevent it from retracting up into the superior mediastinum. Alternatively, a 2-0 silk through the anterior aspect of the trachea can be placed to assist with traction. Insert the first stitch for the tracheal anastomosis through the recipient trachea at the 3 o'clock position. Access to the recipient tracheal stump can then be maintained with gentle traction on this suture. Complete the division of the membranous part of the trachea and excise the recipient carina. The line of cut on the membranous trachea should be convex downward to leave an excess of tissue on the recipient trachea, because it tends to retract once traction has been released.

Step 21. Readying the donor heart-lung bloc. Partially wrap the donor heart-lung bloc in a cold, wet laparotomy pad and steady it in the anatomic orientation on the recipient's epigastrium (Fig. 7-18).

Step 22. Posterior portion of tracheal anastomosis. After placing a 3-0 polypropylene suture in the recipient trachea, begin the membranous part of the tracheal anastomosis. After making the first two or three passes of this running suture, lower the donor heart-lung bloc inside the recipient's chest cavity. Support the weight of the donor organs by placing your right hand behind the donor heart. Use your left hand to maneuver the right donor lung through the pericardial window into the right pleural cavity. At the same time the assistant gently takes up the slack on the two ends of the running suture to approximate the donor carina and the recipient trachea. Maneuver the left lung through the corresponding pericardial window into the left pleural cavity. Finally, lower the donor heart into the pericardial cavity. At this stage, check the orientation of each lobe of the lungs to ensure that they have not been rotated around their axis during passage through the respective pericardial windows. Traction of the donor aorta anteriorly and

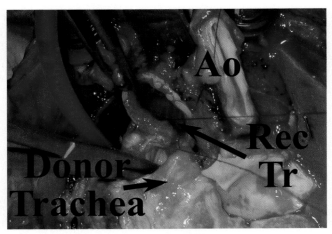

Figure 7-19. Rec Tr, recipient trachea.

inferiorly provides exposure for the completion of the tracheal anastomosis. Place the row of running suture for the membranous part of the trachea from the inside of the trachea, moving from the patient's left side to the right (Fig. 7-19).

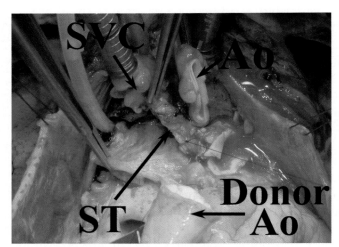

Figure 7-20. ST, peritracheal soft tissue; Ao, recipient aorta; donor Ao, donor aorta; SVC, superior vena cava.

Step 23. Anterior portion of tracheal anastomosis. Continue the same suture onto the cartilaginous part of the trachea, and place the anterior row of suture from the outside of the trachea. Once the tracheal anastomosis is complete, loosely approximate the peritracheal soft tissue surrounding the donor and recipient airways with a running 4-0 polypropylene suture to cover the anastomosis (Fig. 7-20).

Step 24. Initial ventilation of implanted lungs. Any blood that collects in the airways during the tracheal anastomosis should be aspirated by the anesthesiologist using flexible bronchoscopy. The lungs are gently reinflated and ventilated with a tidal volume of 5 mL/kg from this point onwards. If possible, ventilation occurs using room air. The oxygen content of the inspired air is increased only if necessary to wean the patient from CPB. Ventilation does not usually interfere with the remainder of the implant operation.

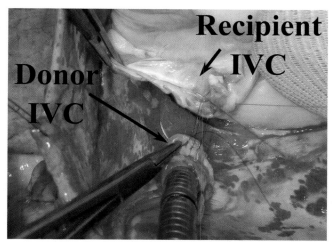

Figure 7-21.

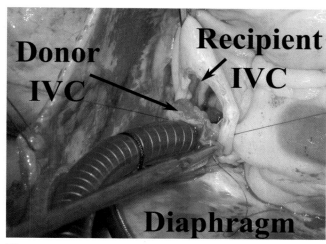

Figure 7-22.

Step 25. Inferior vena cava anastomosis. Once the tracheal anastomosis has been completed, turn your attention to the IVC. Since the IVC lies deep within the pericardial cavity, access can be difficult. Displacing the heart through the left pericardial window into the left pleural cavity enhances exposure for this anastomosis. Perform the IVC anastomosis with an extra-long 3-0 polypropylene running suture beginning with the posterior wall (Fig. 7-21).

Step 26. Inferior vena cava anastomosis (2). At this stage, there always appears to be a substantial size mismatch between the donor IVC and the recipient IVC. The nylon tape that is used to encircle and snare the recipient IVC around the venous cannula causes this apparent size mismatch. By using many very closely placed sutures with the running stitch, the IVC anastomosis can be completed with little difficulty. The IVC anastomosis continues around the anterior aspect of the vessel until completed (Fig. 7-22).

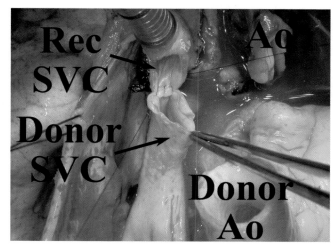

Figure 7-23. Rec SVC, recipient superior vena cava; Ao, recipient aorta.

Step 27. SVC anastomosis. Return the heart to the pericardial cavity and complete the SVC anastomosis using a 4-0 polypropylene running suture, taking care to avoid torsion between the donor and recipient SVC (Fig. 7-23).

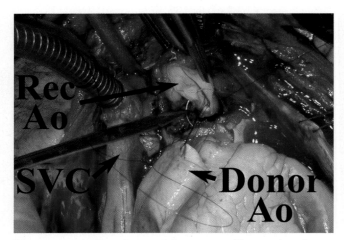

Figure 7-24. Rec Ao, recipient aorta; Donor Ao, donor aorta.

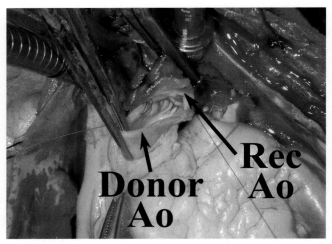

Figure 7-25. Rec Ao, recipient aorta; Donor Ao, donor aorta.

Step 28. Aortic anastomosis. Leave this suture untied for subsequent de-airing of the right atrium just before release of the aortic cross-clamp. After this step, the pulmonary artery catheter may be advanced if one is desired. Gradual warming of the patient to 37°C begins. Perform the aortic anastomosis with a 4-0 polypropylene running suture (Figs. 7-24 and 7-25).

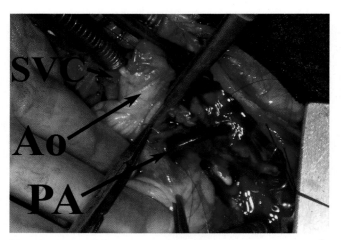

Figure 7-26. PA, pneumoplegia cannulation site in pulmonary trunk.

Step 29. De-airing of the heart. The patient is placed steeply head-down in preparation for de-airing of the heart. Remove the nylon tapes around the venae cavae and partially unclamp the venous circuit to allow filling of the heart. The right atrium is thoroughly de-aired through the SVC anastomosis before the suture is tied. Next, the right ventricle is de-aired through the pneumoplegia site in the donor pulmonary trunk (Fig. 7-26).

Step 30. Reperfusion of the heart-lung bloc. Increase the tidal volume of the ventilator to 10 mL/kg. As more blood is allowed to flow across the pulmonary bed, de-airing of the left heart can be accomplished through the vent opening on the tip of the left atrial appendage as well as the cardioplegia site in the donor aor-

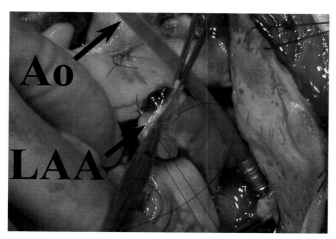

Figure 7-27. LAA, left atrial appendage; Ao, aorta.

tic root. Remove the aortic cross-clamp and begin reperfusion of the implanted organ. Controlled reperfusion of transplanted lungs has been shown to reduce leukocyte sequestration and endothelial permeability in the pulmonary graft. It is therefore advisable to maintain the mean PA pressure below 10 mm Hg for the first 10 minutes and below 20 mm Hg for the next 10 minutes during the initial reperfusion period.

Step 31. Completion of de-airing. At this stage, we routinely start an isoprenaline infusion (0.02 μg/kg/min) and a dopamine infusion (5 μg/kg/min) to decrease pulmonary vascular resistance and to increase cardiac contractility. Further de-airing of the heart is undertaken before the de-airing sites in the pulmonary trunk, the left atrial appendage, and the aortic root are closed in turn with 4-0 polypropylene sutures. Figure 7-27 shows the left atrial appendage being sutured closed after complete de-airing of the transplanted heart.

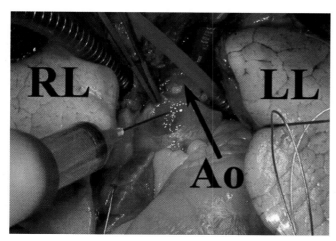

Figure 7-28. LL, left lung; RL, right lung.

Step 32. Completion of de-airing (2). In addition, the aorta can be de-aired with a 21-gauge needle or a cardioplegia cannula attached to a suction catheter (Fig. 7-28).

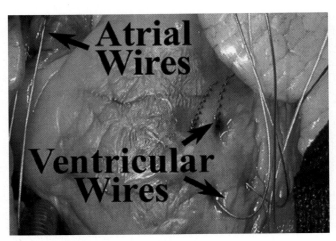

Figure 7-29.

Step 33. Placement of epicardial pacing wires. Secure temporary epicardial pacing wires to the donor right atrium and right ventricle and bring them out through the skin below the incision (Fig. 7-29).

Step 34. Placement of pleural drains and hemostasis. Careful positioning of the chest drains is crucial after heart-lung transplantation to enable early detection of postoperative hemorrhage and to prevent blood from accumulating inside the chest cavity. Insert a pleural drain in the midaxillary line on each side. This is directed toward the posterior costophrenic angle and then along the paravertebral gutter to the apex of the pleural cavity. Cut additional side holes into these drains at the level of the costophrenic angle. Two mediastinal drains are positioned anteriorly, one to lie in the posterior pericardial cavity and the other one retrosternally. The drains are connected to drain bottles with underwater seal and placed on suction of 7 kPa. When normothermia is achieved, the patient can be weaned off CPB. Avoid overdistension of the heart at this stage. When the venous cannulas have been removed, reverse residual heparin with protamine sulfate (3 mg/kg). Clotting factors and platelets are routinely administered because postoperative hemorrhage is a common complication of heart-lung transplant. Finally, remove the aortic cannula and ensure hemostasis before closing the sternotomy.

Section IV
Liver Transplantation

Chapter 8

Adult Cadaveric Liver Transplantation

■ **Carlos E. Marroquin, M.D.**

■ **Bradley H. Collins, M.D.**

■ **J. Elizabeth Tuttle-Newhall, M.D.**

■ **Paul C. Kuo, M.D., M.B.A.**

Department of Surgery, Duke University Medical Center, Durham, NC

INTRODUCTION

The clinical application of liver transplantation grew from experimental techniques employed in dogs by Moore in Boston and Starzl in Chicago and Denver in 1956. Starzl first attempted replacement of a diseased liver in a patient with biliary atresia in 1963. Despite extensive laboratory successes, this attempt in a small child with multiple prior operations and significant portal hypertension resulted in the intraoperative death of the recipient due to massive hemorrhage. During the ensuing years, isolated attempts at liver transplantation were made at several institutions. However, these efforts did not result in any long-term survivors, and an unofficial moratorium on clinical liver transplantation resulted. The development of antilymphocyte serum in 1966 improved graft survival, and Starzl performed the first successful long-term liver transplant procedure in 1967. Barriers to solid organ transplantation included the lack of social and legal reform measures allowing use of organs for transplantation from donors after declaration of brain death. The Harvard Ad-Hoc Committee Report on Brain Death in 1968 gained public support, and soon afterward the courts provided a legal definition of the concept of death and cessation of brain function. However, consistent long-term success had to await the evolution of more refined immunosuppression techniques.

With the introduction of cyclosporine A in 1979, liver and other solid organ transplantation began to emerge as a viable treatment for end-state organ disease.

The National Institutes of Health Consensus Development Conference on Liver Transplantation in 1983 further validated the field of liver transplantation as a therapeutic option for patients with end-stage liver disease. Liver transplant centers began to develop worldwide, and successful liver transplantation became the expectation. Other significant advances included the development of University of Wisconsin (UW) solution by Belzer for preservation of hepatic allografts, which safely extended preservation times and allowed sharing of organs from great distances, thus relaxing logistic constraints. Refinement of anesthetic and perioperative management of the liver transplant recipient further improved the operative results. Shaw and colleagues introduced a venovenous bypass circuit that allowed a smoother hemodynamic course during interruption of the venous return circulation to the heart, enabling the operation to proceed in a more controlled fashion. Other innovations included the development of the piggyback technique, which allows preservation of the recipient vena cava, and the development of the immunosuppressive agent tacrolimus in 1986. The most recent development in liver transplantation has been the practical application of living-donor liver transplantation to children and adults awaiting liver transplantation.

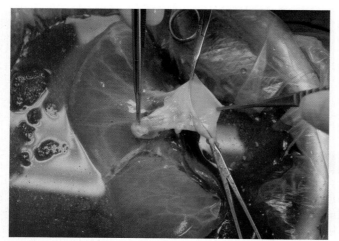

Figure 8-1.

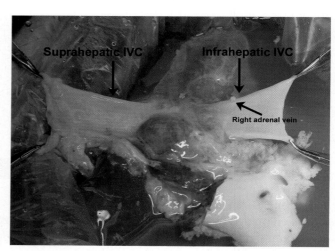

Figure 8-2.

Step 1. Back-table preparation of the liver allograft. Remove the residual diaphragm from the bare area of the right lobe and the suprahepatic inferior vena cava. Trim the suprahepatic inferior vena cava (IVC) to the appropriate length. Identify and ligate the orifices of the three phrenic vein branches. Inspect the hepatic veins to ensure patency and lack of injury (Fig. 8-1)

Step 2. Back-table preparation of the liver allograft (2). Inspect the IVC along its retrohepatic length to locate potential sites of hemorrhage following reperfusion. Identify the right adrenal vein along the lateral margin of the infrahepatic IVC and ligate it. Excise the residual right adrenal gland. The infrahepatic IVC can be further lengthened by ligating small caudate and right lobe venous branches (Fig. 8-2).

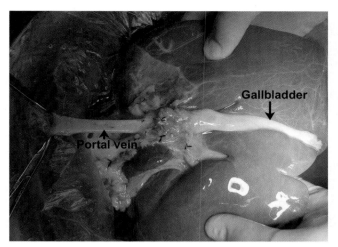

Figure 8-3.

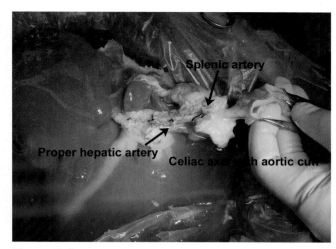

Figure 8-4.

Step 3. Back-table preparation of the liver allograft (3). Dissect the portal vein away from surrounding hilar adventitial tissue to maximize length. Ligate the coronary vein branch. A replaced right hepatic artery may lie posterior to the portal vein or common bile duct (Fig. 8-3).

Step 4. Back-table preparation of the liver allograft (4). Remove residual muscle and ganglial tissue from the aortic cuff, celiac axis, and proper hepatic artery. Identify the splenic and left gastric artery branches and ligate them. The dissection terminates at the gastroduodenal artery branch. Use a 1- or 2-mm coronary dilator to gently probe the right and left hepatic arteries to confirm patency (Fig. 8-4).

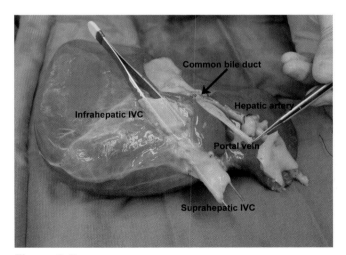

Figure 8-5.

Step 5. Completion of back-table preparation of liver allograft. Upon completion of back-table preparation, the major vascular structures are readily identifiable. Minimize dissection around the common bile duct to avoid devascularization. The gallbladder can now be removed, if desired (Fig. 8-5).

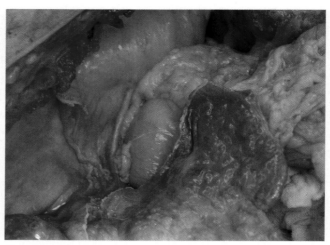

Figure 8-6.

Step 6. Incision and retractor placement for exposure. The patient is positioned with both arms extended to allow ready access. The left chest, abdomen, left groin, and left axilla are prepared and draped. This allows use of venovenous bypass, if needed. Make a generous bilateral subcostal incision with an upward midline extension. In the presence of severe portal hypertension, large portosystemic collaterals may be found in the subcutaneous tissue. Divide the falciform ligament to the level of the suprahepatic vena cava. Fixed retraction devices are critical for achieving maximal exposure. Three blades are placed on the left and right costal margins and the xiphoid process for cephalad retraction. Later, two additional retractor blades are placed on the stomach and hepatic flexure for caudal exposure.

Step 7. Mobilization of the left lobe. Divide the left triangular ligament medially to the IVC. Avoid injuring the phrenic veins or the underlying stomach (Fig. 8-6).

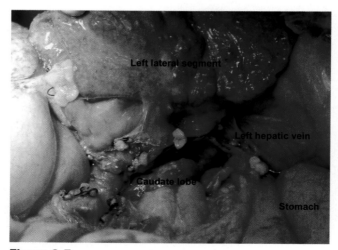

Figure 8-7.

Step 8. Division of the gastrohepatic ligament. Divide the gastrohepatic ligament from the porta hepatis to the area of the left hepatic vein. Frequently, this must be performed between clamps and ligatures. A replaced left hepatic artery may be located in this ligament (Fig. 8-7).

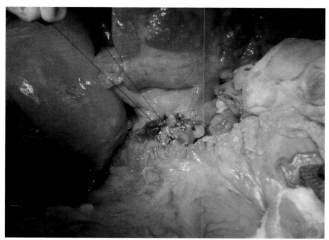

Figure 8-8.

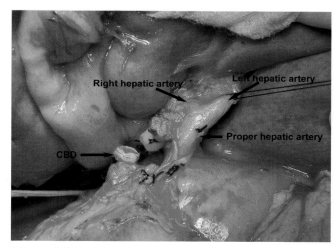

Figure 8-9.

Step 9. Porta hepatis dissection. The dissection in the porta hepatis proceeds using clamps and ties or electrocautery. Varices may require suture ligature. Palpate the hepatic artery to determine its anatomic course. Take care to determine the presence of a replaced right hepatic artery. Palpate the portal vein posteriorly to ascertain the presence of clot or obliteration (Fig. 8-8).

Step 10. Porta hepatis dissection (2). Divide the common bile duct (CBD) high in the hilum to maintain adequate recipient length. Dissect the proper hepatic artery to its bifurcation into a standard right and left hepatic artery (Fig. 8-9).

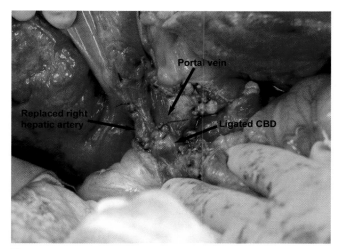

Figure 8-10.

Step 11. Porta hepatis dissection, alternative anatomy. The common bile duct has been ligated, exposing a replaced right hepatic artery. Posteriorly, note the portal vein (Fig. 8-10).

Step 12. Porta hepatis dissection (3). The common bile duct and hepatic artery have been ligated. Handle the artery with care to avoid dissection with ligation. Circumferentially clear the portal vein of surrounding fibrous tissue. The cirrhotic

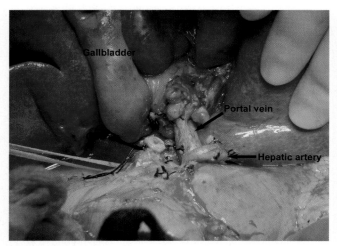

Figure 8-11.

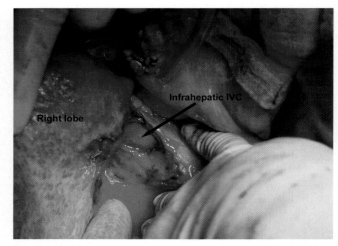

Figure 8-12.

liver has shrunken away from the portal vein bifurcation to expose the right and left portal vein branches (Fig. 8-11).

Step 13. Mobilization of the right lobe and exposure of infrahepatic IVC. Mobilize the right lobe of the liver by superior and inferior division of the right triangular ligament. This maneuver is frequently associated with brisk variceal bleeding from retroperitoneal collaterals. Avoid tearing the ligament when retracting the right lobe. After full mobilization of the right hepatic lobe, divide the peritoneum overlying the infrahepatic IVC and encircle the vessel. In a similar fashion, encircle the suprahepatic IVC (Fig. 8-12). Two alternative approaches will be described, the "piggyback" with recipient caval preservation and the "in-continuity" removal of recipient cava.

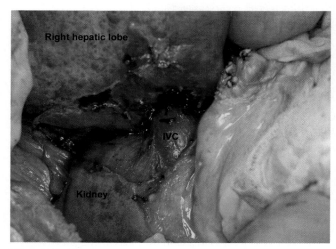

Figure 8-13.

Step 14. Division of hepatic veins draining right hepatic lobe (piggyback technique). Dissect the right lobe free from the anterior surface of the recipient vena cava using gentle blunt technique. Proceed in a cephalad fashion to the level of the main hepatic veins. Clamp, divide, and ligate perforating veins. Oversew larger veins against the cava using figure-of-eight sutures (Fig. 8-13).

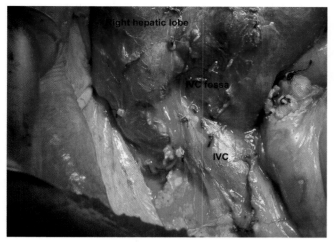

Figure 8-14.

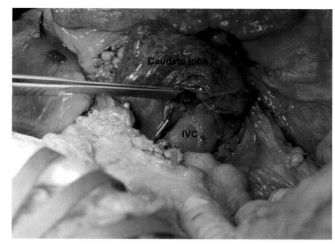

Figure 8-15.

Step 15. Division of hepatic veins draining right hepatic lobe (piggyback technique) (2) (Fig. 8-14).

Step 16. Division of hepatic veins draining caudate lobe (piggyback technique). Dissect the caudate lobe away from the anterior surface of the vena cava. This is typically performed from the left side of the recipient and proceeds in a cephalad fashion. In some cases, the caudate may appear to encircle the vena cava. This connecting bridge of liver tissue can be divided on the right to unwrap the caudate. Alternatively, the caudate may be divided on the left to leave the posterior bridge of caudate in place (Fig. 8-15).

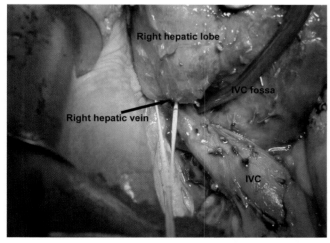

Figure 8-16.

Step 17. Isolation and division of right hepatic vein (piggyback technique). After dividing all secondary hepatic veins from the right and caudate lobes, isolate the right hepatic vein and encircle it with a vessel loop. Avoid injury to the right hepatic vein, as it is frequently fragile, large, and broad-based. Divide the right hepatic vein with a 2.5-mm stapling device (Fig. 8-16).

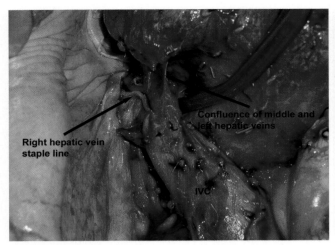

Figure 8-17.

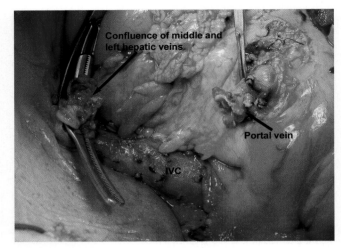

Figure 8-18.

Step 18. Completion of vena caval dissection (piggyback technique). After division of the right hepatic vein, the confluence of the middle and left hepatic veins is visible. Connect the recipient liver to the portal vein and hepatic veins only (Fig. 8-17).

Step 19. Clamping of portal vein and hepatic veins (piggyback technique). Place vascular clamps across the portal vein and confluence of the middle and left hepatic veins. Divide these vessels to maintain maximal length in the recipient. Remove the liver from the operative field. The common wall between the middle and left hepatic veins will be divided and anastomosed to the donor suprahepatic IVC. The piggyback technique maintains vena caval patency and venous return from the lower portion of the body. Inspect the area of the vena cava and adrenal gland for bleeding sites (Fig. 8-18).

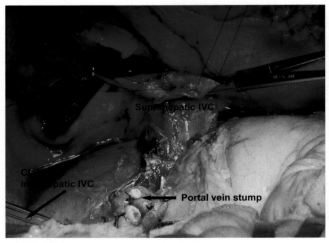

Figure 8-19.

Step 20. Clamping of portal vein, suprahepatic and infrahepatic vena cava (in-continuity technique). Alternatively, the recipient liver may be removed with the retrohepatic portion of the vena cava. In this instance, clamps are placed across the suprahepatic and infrahepatic vena cava and portal vein. The recipient liver with accompanying vena cava is then removed (Fig. 8-19).

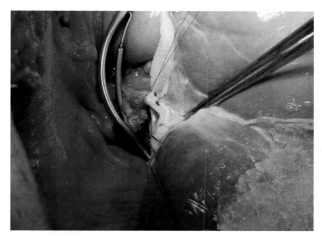

Figure 8-20.

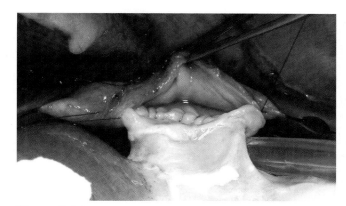

Figure 8-21.

Step 21. Donor liver and upper caval anastomosis. Bring the new donor liver onto the operative field. Place corner stitches of 3-0 polypropylene between the donor suprahepatic cava and the recipient cava, either the confluence of the middle and left hepatic veins (piggyback) or the entire suprahepatic vena caval orifice (in-continuity) (Fig. 8-20).

Step 22. Suprahepatic caval anastomosis. Tie the corner stitch opposite the operating surgeon. Anastomose the posterior walls using a vertical mattress technique to evert the adventitial layer; however, a simple running stitch is also acceptable. Avoid excessive purse-stringing of the anastomosis (Fig. 8-21).

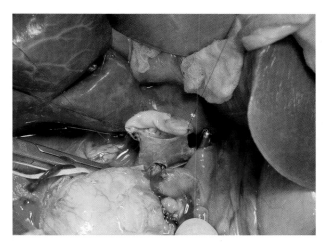

Figure 8-22.

Step 23. Infrahepatic caval anastomosis (in-continuity technique). If the in-continuity technique is used, continue with the infrahepatic caval anastomosis by placing 4-0 polypropylene corner stitches between the donor and recipient infrahepatic cavae. Tie the corner stitch opposite the operating surgeon. Anastomose the posterior walls using a vertical mattress technique to evert the adventitial layer; however, a simple running stitch is also acceptable. Avoid excessive purse-stringing of the anastomosis (Fig. 8-22).

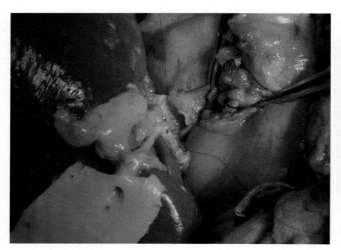

Figure 8-23.

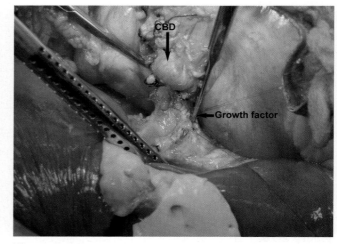

Figure 8-24.

Step 24. Portal vein anastomosis. Trim the donor and recipient portal veins to avoid redundancy. Releasing tension from the cephalad and caudal retractors can be useful. Perform the portal vein anastomosis with two corner stitches of 5-0 polypropylene suture. Anastomose the posterior walls using a vertical mattress technique to evert the adventitial layer; however, a simple running stitch is also acceptable (Fig. 8-23).

Step 25. Portal vein anastomosis. Before completing the anastomosis, transiently open the portal vein clamp to flush out any thrombus. Then tie the suture with an "air-knot," or growth factor, corresponding to approximately one-third the diameter of the portal vein to avoid purse-stringing of the anastomosis (Fig. 8-24).

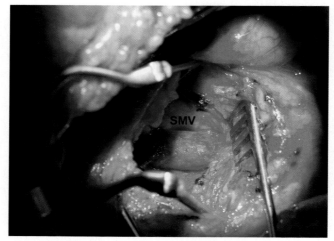

Figure 8-25.

Step 26. Alternative portal venous reconstruction: superior mesenteric vein interposition graft. In the setting of a thrombosed or obliterated portal vein, a superior mesenteric vein graft can be performed using donor iliac vein. The lesser sac is entered and the lower peritoneal edge of the pancreas is incised. The superior mesenteric vein is identified and isolated for a length of 2 to 3 cm (Fig. 8-25).

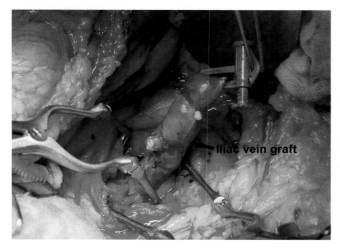

Figure 8-26.

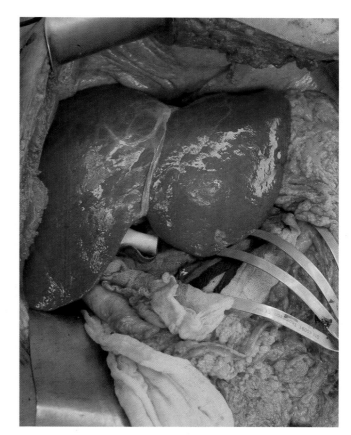

Figure 8-27.

Step 27. Alternative portal venous reconstruction: superior mesenteric vein interposition graft (2). Identify the distal and proximal orientation of the donor vein graft. Anastomose the donor iliac vein in an end-to-side fashion to the superior mesenteric artery using 6-0 polypropylene suture. Tunnel the graft under the stomach and anterior to the pancreas to the area of the hilum of the donor liver. Perform the anastomosis as previously described. It is preferable to perform the superior mesenteric vein interposition graft before beginning the hepatectomy and hilar dissection (Fig. 8-26).

Step 28. Flushing. If you are using the piggyback technique, flush the remaining preservation solution from the new liver via the donor infrahepatic cava. Release the portal vein clamp and flush out approximately 300 mL of blood through the donor infrahepatic vena cava. Then clamp the donor infrahepatic cava and release the suprahepatic vena cava clamp. Staple the infrahepatic cava closed.

If using the in-continuity technique, place a large-bore catheter in the infrahepatic caval anastomosis before tying the suture. Release the portal vein clamp and flush out approximately 300 mL of blood through the catheter in the infrahepatic vena cava. Then tie the donor infrahepatic caval suture after removal of the catheter, and simultaneously release the suprahepatic vena cava clamp.

Step 29. Liver reperfusion. Following hepatic reperfusion, inspect all the anastomoses for bleeding (Fig. 8-27).

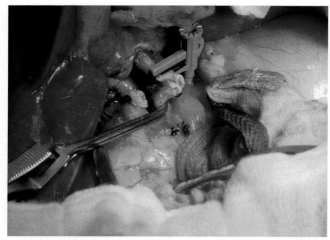

Figure 8-28.

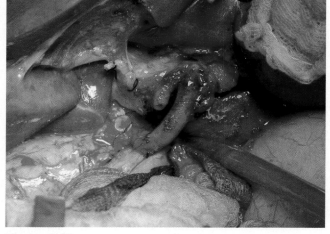

Figure 8-29.

Step 30. Hepatic artery anastomosis. Perform an end-to-end anastomosis between the donor proper hepatic artery and the recipient hepatic artery. Fashion the donor artery into an appropriate Carrel patch at the level of the celiac axis or the splenic artery. Use 6-0 or 7-0 polypropylene suture for the anastomosis (Fig. 8-28).

Step 31. Hepatic artery anastomosis. Before completion of the anastomosis, flush the recipient artery to remove thrombus. A palpable thrill should be palpable in the donor vessel following the anastomosis (Fig. 8-29).

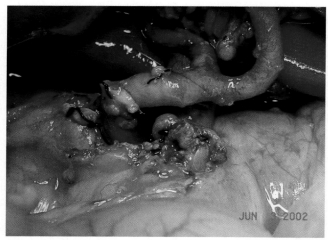

Figure 8-30.

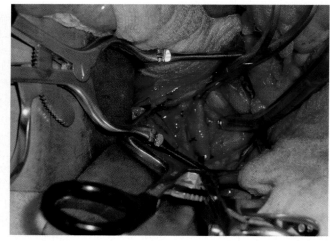

Figure 8-31.

Step 32. Hepatic artery anastomosis (2) (Fig. 8-30).

Step 33. Hepatic artery anastomosis using an aortic conduit. If the recipient artery is unsuitable, an arterial graft based on the infrarenal aorta can be constructed using donor iliac artery. Isolate the infrarenal aorta lateral to the ligament of Treitz (Fig. 8-31).

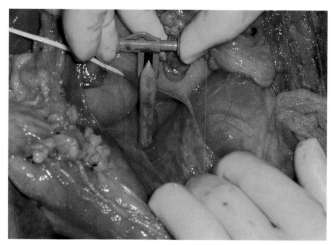

Figure 8-32.

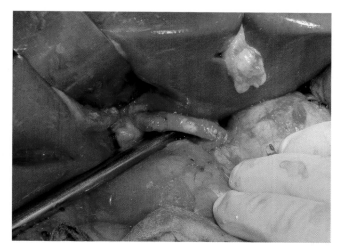

Figure 8-33.

Step 34. Hepatic artery anastomosis using an aortic conduit (2). Anastomose the donor iliac artery to the side of the infrarenal aorta (Fig. 8-32).

Step 35. Hepatic artery anastomosis using an aortic conduit (3). Tunnel the conduit through the transverse mesocolon lateral to the ligament of Treitz and under the stomach to the area of the hepatic hilum to complete the hepatic arterial anastomosis (Fig. 8-33).

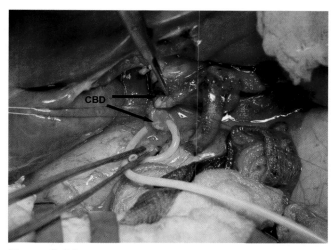

Figure 8-34.

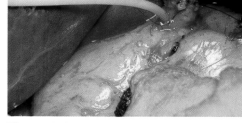

Figure 8-35.

Step 36. Choledochocholedochostomy. Remove the gallbladder. Place a T-tube with its exit site through the recipient common bile duct. Close the exit site with a 5-0 PDS purse-string suture. Control bleeding from the donor bile duct using suture ligatures. Perform a duct-to-duct anastomosis using interrupted 5-0 PDS sutures. Upon completion of the anastomosis, inject dilute saline solution of methylene blue through the T-tube to check for leakage (Fig. 8-34).

Step 37. Choledochocholedochostomy (2) (Fig. 8-35)

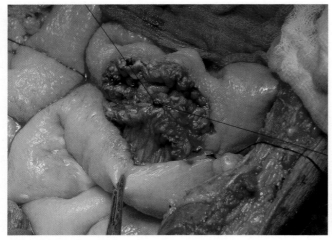

Figure 8-36.

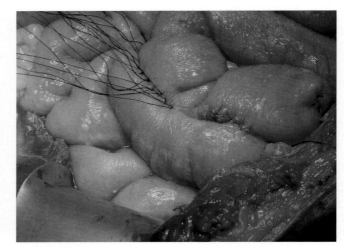

Figure 8-37.

Step 38. Roux-en-Y choledochojejunostomy. In the absence of a suitable recipient common bile duct or primary sclerosing cholangitis, construct a Roux-en-Y choledochojejunostomy. Select a suitable length of jejunum and divide the bowel and mesentery using a stapling device. Measure a 40-cm length of the Roux limb. Construct a side-to-side jejunojejunostomy using a two-layer hand-sewn technique. Close the mesenteric defect (Fig. 8-36).

Step 39. Roux-en-Y choledochojejunostomy (2) (Fig. 8-37).

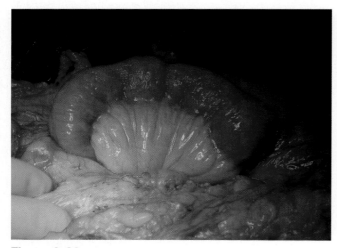

Figure 8-38.

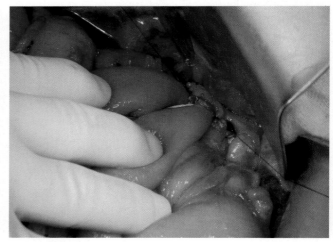

Figure 8-39.

Step 40. Roux-en-Y choledochojejunostomy (3). Place the Roux limb in a retrocolic position (Fig. 8-38).

Step 41. Choledochojejunal biliary anastomosis. Perform the bile duct anastomosis over a biliary stent with an interrupted technique using 5-0 or 6-0 PDS suture. Upon completion of the anastomosis, inject dilute saline solution of methylene blue through the stent to check for leakage (Fig. 8-39).

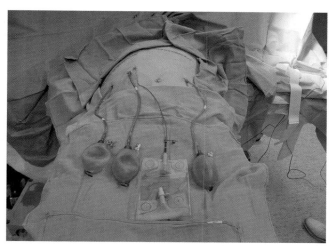

Figure 8-40.

Step 42. Completion of the liver transplant. Close the abdominal fascia using an interrupted technique. Place three drains: over the right lobe, left lobe, and near the biliary anastomosis. Bring the biliary drain out through a separate site (Fig. 8-40).

Chapter 9

Adult Living-Donor Liver Transplantation

- **Lynt B. Johnson, M.D.**
- **Reena C. Jha, M.D.***
- **Amy D. Lu, M.D.**

Department of Surgery; *Department of Radiology, Georgetown University Hospital, Washington, D.C.

- **James J. Pomposelli, M.D., Ph.D.**
- **Elizabeth A. Pomfret, M.D., Ph.D.**

Department of Surgery, Lahey Clinic Medical Center, Burlington, MA

INTRODUCTION

The living-donor right hepatectomy is an operation that carries significant risk for the donor. Unlike other operations, there are no direct physical benefits to the donor. The potential morbidity and mortality is considerably higher than the risk for living-donor kidney removal. In most series the overall complication rate approaches 25%, while the mortality rate is approximately 0.25%. The donor operation consists of a formal right hepatectomy. Donor graft volume is calculated by volumetric analysis using magnetic resonance imaging or spiral computed tomography images. Donor graft weight should equal approximately 1% of recipient body weight to ensure good graft function. Recipients without portal hypertension may do satisfactorily with a graft:weight ratio as low as 0.8%. Preoperative volumetric assessment and topographic planning are paramount to a successful resection.

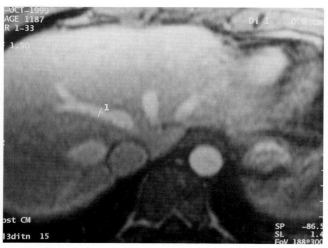

Figure 9-1.

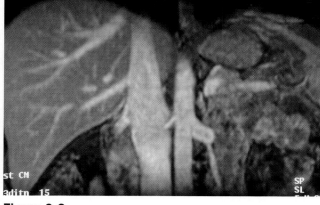

Figure 9-2.

Step 1. MRI of the hepatic vasculature. Axial postcontrast imaging shows the hepatic venous anatomy at the dome of the liver and shows a 1-cm branch of the middle hepatic vein, which drains segment 8 of the liver (Fig. 9-1).

Step 2. MRI of the hepatic vasculature (2). Coronal postcontrast imaging of the liver shows the main right hepatic vein as well as two accessory hepatic veins; one of them is less than 3 mm and the other is more than 5 mm, which requires re-anastomosis in the recipient (Fig. 9-2).

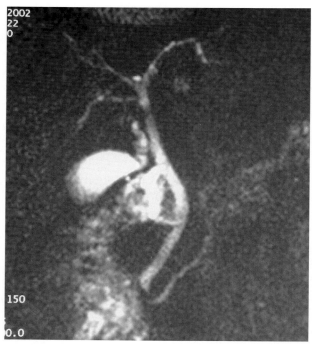

Figure 9-3.

Step 3. Magnetic resonance cholangiopancreatography (MRCP). Coronal MRCP imaging shows an accessory right hepatic duct and an otherwise normal biliary tree (Fig. 9-3).

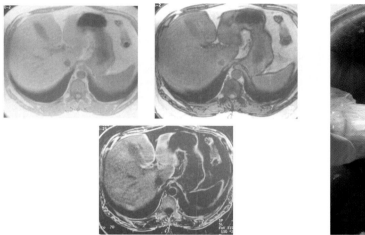

Figure 9-4.

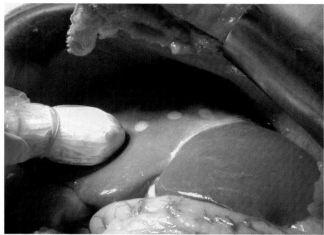

Figure 9-5.

Step 4. MRI for detection of fatty infiltration. Hepatic steatosis is an exclusion criterion for living liver donation. The use of combined in-phase and out-of-phase T1-weighted images allows detection of fatty infiltration, with loss of signal seen on the liver parenchyma compared to the spleen on the out-of-phase images. Subtraction images can be particularly helpful to detect subtle changes of fatty infiltration, with the out-of-phase images subtracted from the in-phase images. Any regions of increased signal on the subtraction images support the presence of parenchymal fatty infiltration (Fig. 9-4).

Step 5. Intraoperative ultrasound (IOUS). IOUS is used to demarcate the line of transection. Locate the middle hepatic vein and mark it using surface cautery. This produces a characteristic artifact, with a shadow seen deep to the cautery site (Fig. 9-5).

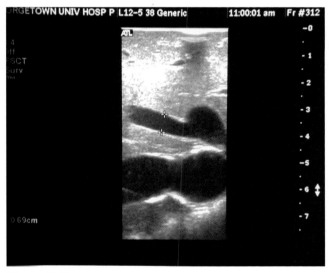

Figure 9-6.

Step 6. IOUS (2). Locate branches of the middle hepatic vein that are in the line of transection; if they are sizable (greater than 5 mm), preserve them. Evaluate for accessory right hepatic veins. The line of transection is 1 cm to the right of the middle hepatic vein (Fig. 9-6).

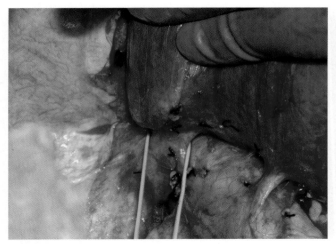

Figure 9-7.

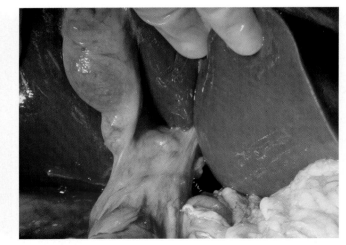

Figure 9-8.

Step 7. Retrohepatic vena cava, main, and inferior hepatic veins. Divide the right triangular ligament and rotate the right hepatic lobe medially to expose the vena cava. Ligate and divide small branches from the vena cava to the right lobe. Preserve the right hepatic vein and any substantial inferior hepatic veins (more than 5 mm) (Fig. 9-7).

Step 8. Porta hepatis. Expose the porta hepatis and divide the peritoneum overlying the hilar structures. Dissect the gallbladder away from the liver and remove it. An intraoperative cholangiogram can be performed at this time to further delineate the biliary tree (Fig. 9-8).

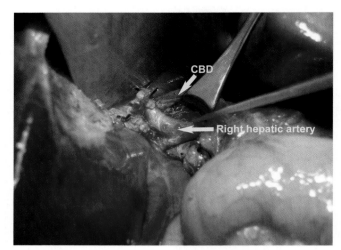

Figure 9-9.

Step 9. Hepatic artery. Trace the right hepatic artery as it passes behind the common bile duct. Using a vein retractor, lift the common bile duct to expose the right branch of the hepatic artery (Fig. 9-9).

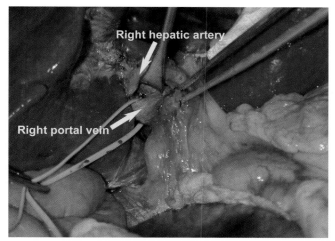

Figure 9-10.

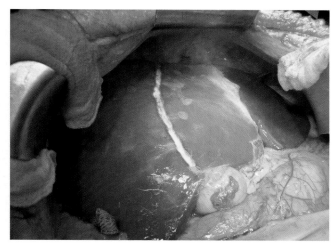

Figure 9-11.

Step 10. Portal vein. Dissect the portal vein from the surrounding adventitial tissue. Insert the vein retractor beneath the right hepatic artery to further expose the bifurcation of the portal vein. A small posterior caudate branch is usually identified and ligated before encircling the right portal vein with a vessel loop (Fig. 9-10).

Step 11. Parenchymal transection. With the argon beam coagulator, mark the proposed division line 1 cm to the right of the middle hepatic vein. Divide a small portion of the right half of the caudate lobe to avoid biliary devascularization. Pass an umbilical tape beneath the liver to the left of the right hepatic vein and though the divided caudate and finally though the bifurcation of the portal vein. The umbilical tape guides the transection as it proceeds through the parenchyma (Fig. 9-11).

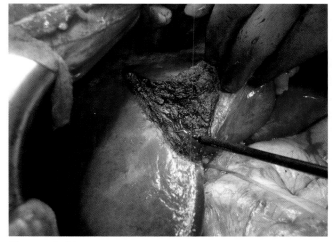

Figure 9-12.

Step 12. Harmonic scalpel. Use the harmonic scalpel to minimize blood loss during the parenchymal transection. The parenchymal dissection is performed without vascular occlusion to prevent ischemic damage to the graft (Fig. 9-12).

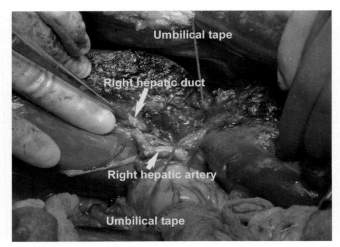

Figure 9-13.

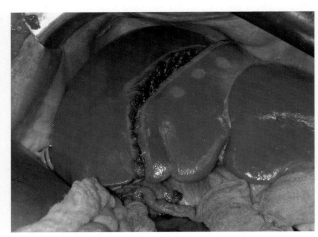

Figure 9-14.

Step 13. Right hepatic duct division. As the dissection nears the hilar plate, transect the right hepatic duct with the scissors, staying close to the transected parenchyma to minimize ischemic injury. Do not use cautery adjacent to the bile duct transection. The forceps identifies the transected right hepatic duct. Often more than one duct is present in the plane of transection. Small (less than 2 mm) posterior ducts may be oversewn when there are prominent right anterior ducts available for reconstruction. In the background, the liver parenchymal transection is nearly complete as the liver hangs on the umbilical tape guide (Fig. 9-13).

Step 14. Completed hepatic transection. The transection of the right lobe is complete. Administer intravenous heparin (70 units/kg). Ligate and divide the right hepatic artery. Then place a clamp across the right branch of the portal vein. Take care not to narrow the left portal vein. Lastly, place a clamp across the right hepatic vein and transect it (Fig. 9-14).

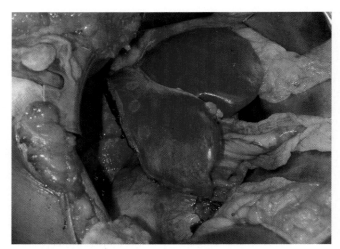

Figure 9-15.

Step 15. Remaining left hepatic lobe. Remove the graft. Oversew the stumps of the right portal vein and hepatic vein. Obtain hemostasis on the cut surface. The left triangular ligament is not disturbed so that the left lobe does not torse following removal of the right lobe (Fig. 9-15).

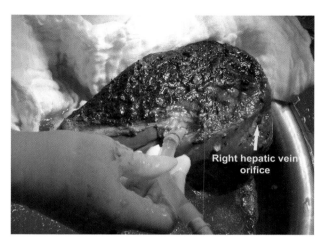

Figure 9-16.

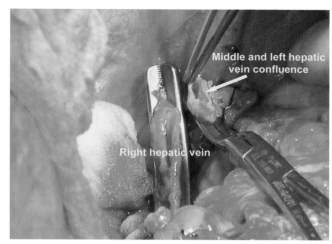

Figure 9-17.

Step 16. Preparation of right lobe graft. Place the right lobe in a basin of iced chilled lactated Ringer's solution. Cannulate the right portal vein and flush it with chilled Belzer's solution. Similarly flush the hepatic artery. Flushing the hepatic duct with preservation solution can often identify transected bile radicals on the parenchymal surface (Fig. 9-16).

Step 17. Recipient procedure. The recipient procedure is performed using a variation of the piggyback technique previously described. The middle and left hepatic veins are oversewn and the donor right hepatic vein is anastomosed to the recipient right hepatic vein.

Step 18. Recipient operation (2). Place clamps across the recipient right hepatic vein and the confluence of the middle and left hepatic veins. Oversew the confluence of the middle and left hepatic veins (Fig. 9-17).

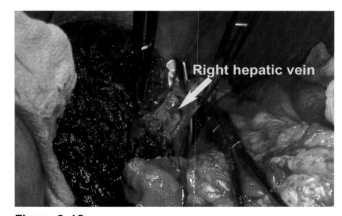

Figure 9-18.

Step 19. Hepatic vein anastomosis. The back wall is completed first. Before completion, flush the graft to remove the perfusate (Fig. 9-18).

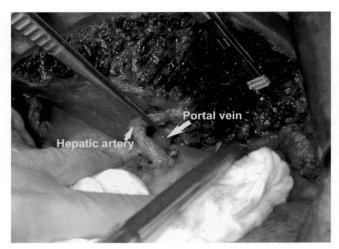

Figure 9-19.

Step 20. Portal vein, hepatic artery anastomosis. Complete the portal vein and hepatic artery anastomoses. The hepatic artery anastomosis is performed with 4.5× magnification. Use fine interrupted suture to complete the arterial anastomosis (Fig. 9-19).

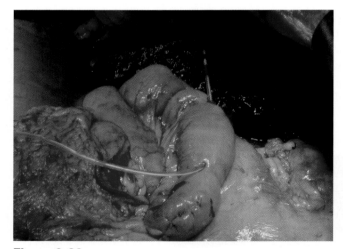

Figure 9-20.

Step 21. Bile duct reconstruction. Construct a Roux-en-Y limb and bring it retrocolic to create an hepaticojejunostomy. Use a 5 Fr pediatric feeding tube as a biliary stent. Then construct the anastomosis with interrupted 5-0 PDS suture over the bile stent (Fig. 9-20).

Chapter 10

Pediatric Living-Donor Liver Transplantation

■ **Jeffrey A. Lowell, M.D.**

■ **Surendra Shenoy, M.D., Ph.D.**

■ **Niraj M. Desai, M.D.**

■ **Martin Jendrisak, M.D.**

■ **Ross W. Shepherd, M.D.**

■ **William C. Chapman, M.D.**

Department of Surgery,
Washington University School of Medicine,
St. Louis, MO

INTRODUCTION

Evaluation of the adult left lateral section liver donor begins after the potential donor contacts the transplant center and volunteers to undergo the procedure. Donors need not be genetically related to the recipient. Altruistic donation, where there is no prior relationship between the donor and recipient, is occurring with increasing frequency. Before beginning the diagnostic testing, ABO blood typing of the donor is established. ABO-compatible donors are given written materials describing the procedure and the likelihood of major and minor complications. They undergo medical evaluation by a medical physician who is not a member of the transplant team. Laboratory testing is then performed, including a complete metabolic profile, liver function tests, serologic tests for hepatitis A, B, and C, and HIV and HTLV III. Magnetic resonance imaging/magnetic resonance angiography (MRI/MRA) or computed tomographic angiography with three-dimensional reconstruction is then performed to determine the arterial and biliary anatomy of the donor liver segment. An accessory left hepatic artery arising from the left gastric artery may pose a problem. Options would include reimplantation of this branch (either end-to-side or side-to-side) into the main left hepatic artery, ligation if it is thought to be inconsequential, or forgoing use of this donor segment.

Portal and biliary anomalies to the left lateral liver segment are very unusual. A preoperative percutaneous liver biopsy may be indicated if the preoperative imaging tests suggest hepatic steatosis.

Living-donor left lateral section liver transplantation from an adult donor to an infant or toddler has many benefits. The procedures can be performed after thorough investigation and determination of the anatomic configurations of both the donor and recipient. Preoperative considerations for the child include recipient size, nutritional status, patency of the portal vein, and the presence of concomitant congenital anomalies. The most common indications for liver transplantation in the infant or toddler are biliary atresia and metabolic inborn errors of metabolism.

Ideally, medical and nutritional support can be provided to the child to allow growth to at least 10 kg. Left lateral section grafts from large adult donors may be difficult to fit into the abdomen of a small newborn, especially if the child's native liver is not enlarged from cholestasis or if significant ascites has not been present. In these situations, a temporary abdominal wall patch may be necessary to close the abdomen after transplantation of the graft. Thrombosis of the portal vein may be identified preoperatively by Doppler ultrasound or MRI/MRA. If thrombosed, a graft to supply portal blood from the superior mesenteric vein may be necessary. A saphenous vein allograft from the living liver donor may be used as an interposition graft. In addition, a saphenous vein allograft may also be necessary if the child's hepatic artery is unusable (i.e., if it is too small, if there is inadequate flow, or if dissection occurs). The upper thigh of the donor should be prepared in case it is necessary to use a saphenous vein graft.

Preoperative evaluation of the recipient should exclude congenital neurologic, cardiac, pulmonary, or renal disease in the child. Psychosocial and financial evaluations of the infant's family should also be conducted to ensure that posttransplantation home care of the child is both adequate and optimized.

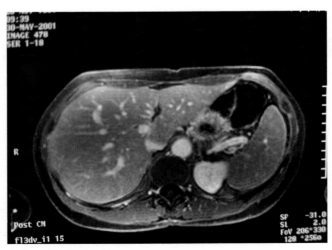

Figure 10-1.

Step 1. CT scan. Preoperative assessment includes tomographic assessment of the liver with either CT or MRI to assess the size/volume of the left lateral section and parenchyma (Fig. 10-1).

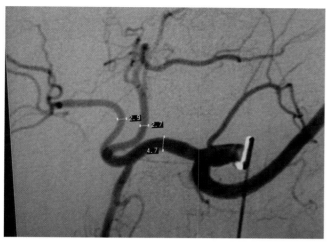

Figure 10-2.

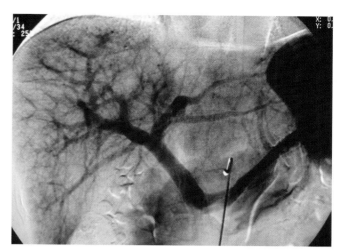

Figure 10-3.

Step 2. Celiac arteriography. Angiography is used to define the arterial and portal anatomy. It is important to evaluate the size of the left hepatic artery. It should be comparable in size to the right hepatic artery (Fig. 10-2).

Step 3. Celiac arteriography (2). Figure 10-3 shows the venous phase of the celiac arteriogram.

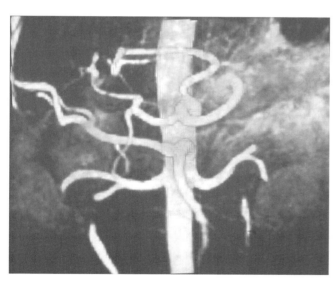

Figure 10-4.

Figure 10-5.

Step 4. Magnetic resonance angiography. MRA can be used as an alternative to conventional arteriography. Three-dimensional reconstruction of the vascular anatomy is possible (Fig. 10-4).

Step 5. Cholangiography. Endoscopic retrograde cholangiography is used to define the biliary anatomy to the left lateral section (Fig. 10-5).

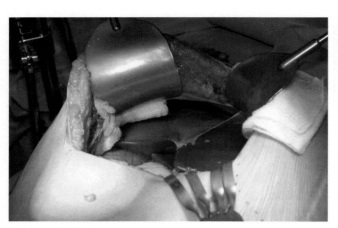

Figure 10-6.

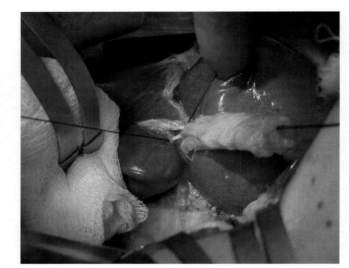

Figure 10-7.

Step 6. Donor incision. The donor procedure begins after a urinary catheter, monitor, and fluid resuscitation intravenous lines are placed and general endotracheal anesthesia is administered. The patient's arms are extended 90 degrees. Make a subcostal incision with a vertical midline extension. The subcostal incision may be extended to the patient's left for added exposure. Use a self-retaining retractor to elevate the rib cage and retract the colon, duodenum, and stomach (Fig. 10-6).

Step 7. Liver mobilization. Divide the round and falciform ligaments and left triangular ligament. Leave a long tie on the round ligament for retraction (Fig. 10-7).

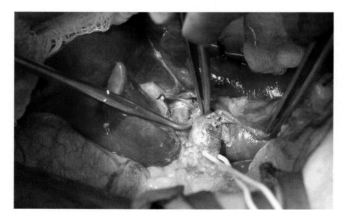

Figure 10-8.

Step 8. Hepatic artery and portal vein. Identify the left hepatic artery branch and trace it to the level of the bifurcation of the main hepatic artery. Divide the portal venous tributaries entering to the right side of the round ligament. Ligating and dividing these branches will bring the left portal vein into clear view (Fig. 10-8).

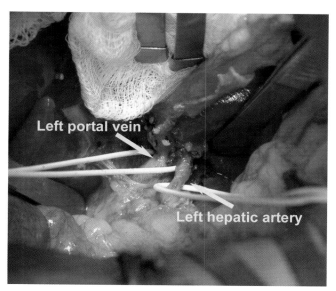

Figure 10-9.

Step 9. Vascular control of left hepatic artery and portal vein. Place elastic vascular tapes around the left portal vein and hepatic artery (Fig. 10-9).

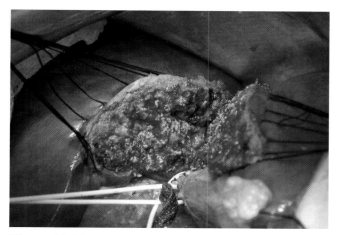

Figure 10-10.

Step 10. Parenchymal dissection. Begin the parenchymal dissection to the right of the falciform ligament after marking the line of resection with electrocautery. Overlapping sutures in the capsule on either side of the line of retraction can aid in retraction and control superficial capsular vessels. The parenchyma can be separated and divided with various techniques, such as hydro- or ultrasonic dissectors. Control vessels with electrocautery or argon beam coagulation. Control larger vessels and small biliary radicals with suture ligature. Also divide the parenchyma bridging the left lateral section and caudate lobe (Fig. 10-10).

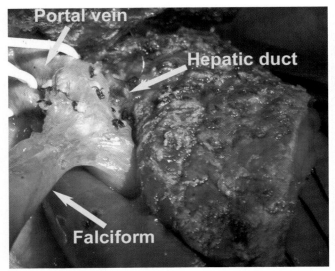

Figure 10-11.

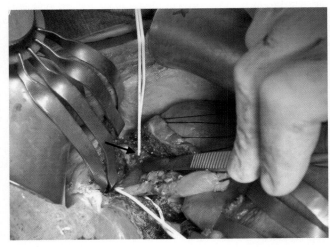

Figure 10-12.

Step 11. Identification and division of bile duct(s). Locate the bile ducts to segments 2 and 3 in the parenchyma just cephalad and anterior to the entrance of the artery and portal vein into the substance of the liver. The ducts may be completely separate, may share a common wall, or may be completely joined at the level that they are divided. Do not use cautery to divide the bile duct(s); rather, use a scissors or scalpel. Leave a suture to mark the duct(s) for later identification (Fig. 10-11).

Step 12. Hepatic vein. The left hepatic vein can be isolated either before the parenchymal dissection or after the parenchyma has been divided up to the level of the hepatic vein. Encircle the left hepatic vein with an elastic vascular tape (arrow, Fig. 10-12).

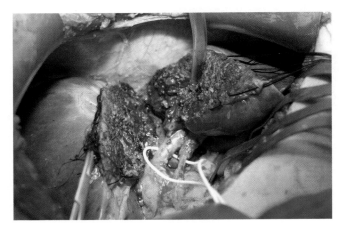

Figure 10-13.

Step 13. Graft ready for removal. The donor left lateral segment is ready for removal (Fig. 10-13).

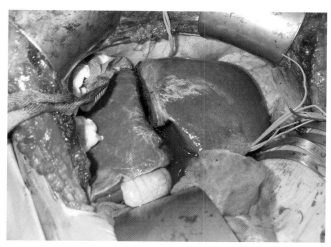

Figure 10-14.

Step 14. Graft ready for removal (2). After communicating with the recipient's operating team, give the patient systemic heparin and place vascular clamps on the left hepatic artery, left portal vein, and left hepatic vein. Then remove the graft and flush it with Belzer solution through the portal vein and then the artery until the effluent is clear. Also back-flush the graft through the hepatic vein (Fig. 10-14).

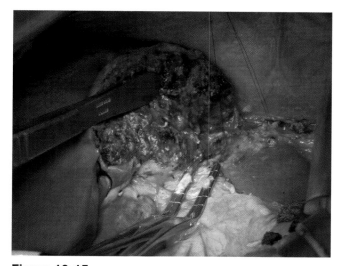

Figure 10-15.

Step 15. Vessels secured. Oversew the openings in the hepatic vein and portal vein and artery with vascular suture. Do not narrow the take-off of the right portal vein. Close the opening in the bile duct(s) with an absorbable monofilament suture. Close the lateral fascia layers in two layers. Close the midline fascia in one layer. Close the dermis with an absorbable subcuticular suture and skin tapes (Fig. 10-15).

Step 16. Recipient positioning. The patient is positioned after induction of general endotracheal anesthesia. All pressure points are well padded, and radial artery catheter, a urinary bladder catheter, and a nasogastric tube are placed. A double-lumen, tunneled Silastic catheter is placed. This can be done through a cutdown of the jugular vein or using a percutaneous technique into the jugular or subclavian vein.

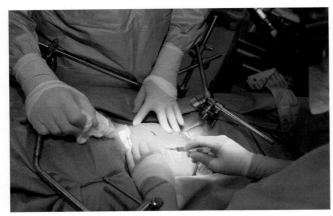

Figure 10-16.

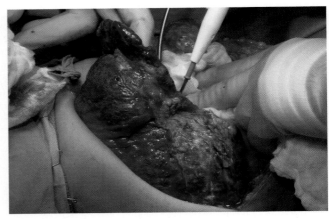

Figure 10-17.

Step 17. Positioning and retractor placement. The infant is repositioned with the arms above the head, and all pressure points are again checked for adequate padding. Thermal warming blankets are used. A self-retaining retractor is used. Make a bilateral subcostal incision, incorporating, if present, the previous incision from the porto-enterostomy (Fig. 10-16).

Step 18. Mobilization of the liver. Open the fascial layers and identify the enlarged, cirrhotic liver. Mobilize it from the adhesions from the previous Kasai procedure (Fig. 10-17).

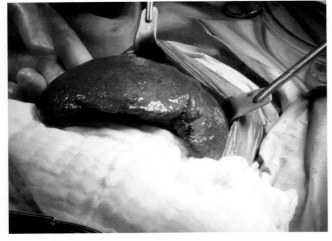

Figure 10-18.

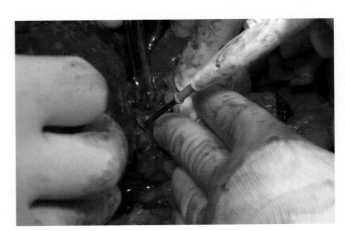

Figure 10-19.

Step 19. Mobilization of the liver (2) (Fig. 10-18).

Step 20. Hepaticojejunostomy taken down. If present, take down the portoenterostomy Roux-en-Y limb from the hilum of the liver and suture the enterostomy closed (Fig. 10-19).

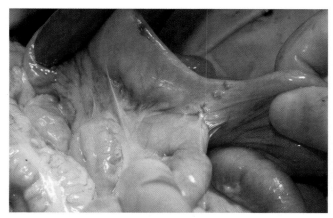

Figure 10-20.

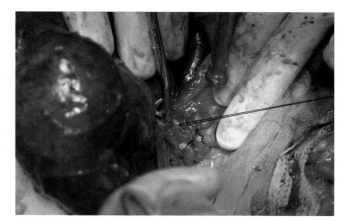

Figure 10-21.

Step 21. Roux-en-Y limb is prepared. Mobilize the Roux-en-Y limb from the surrounding adhesions and free it from where it crosses the transverse mesocolon. Inspect the previous entero-enterostomy and ensure that the Roux-en-Y limb is of adequate length (Fig. 10-20).

Step 22. Hepatic artery identified and mobilized. Individually isolate, ligate, and divide the hepatic artery branches. Divide the gastroduodenal artery. Mobilize the common hepatic artery to the level of the celiac artery (Fig. 10-21).

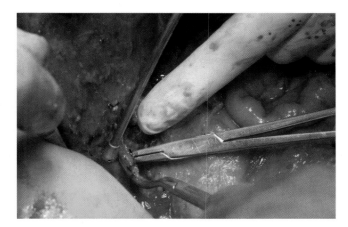

Figure 10-22.

Step 23. Liver mobilized off vena cava. Mobilize the liver off the inferior vena cava. Isolate, ligate, and divide the short hepatic veins connecting the right lobe and caudate lobe with the vena cava. Oversew the vena caval branch stumps with fine vascular suture. With sufficient mobilization of the liver off the vena cava, create a temporary end-to-side portacaval shunt. Place a side-biting clamp on the vena cava and anastomose the portal vein, using a continuous fine vascular suture (Fig. 10-22).

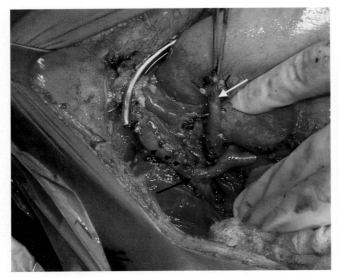

Figure 10-23.

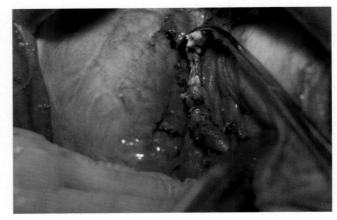

Figure 10-24.

Step 24. Cirrhotic native liver removed. Place a side-biting vascular clamp across the right, middle, and left hepatic veins, and remove the cirrhotic liver. Figure 10-23 shows the clamp across the hepatic veins, the portacaval shunt (black arrow), and the hepatic artery, which has been mobilized to the level of the celiac artery (white arrow). Also noted are the ligated short hepatic veins (small dashed arrow).

Step 25. Replacement of inadequate native vena cava. Occasionally the native, infrahepatic inferior vena cava is atretic or narrow. In this case, consider replacing this segment of vena cava with a vascular interposition graft, such as a cadaveric (blood group-compatible) iliac vein allograft (Fig. 10-24).

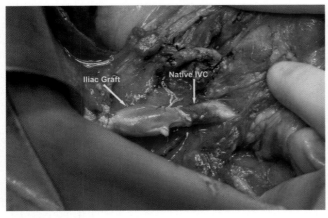

Figure 10-25.

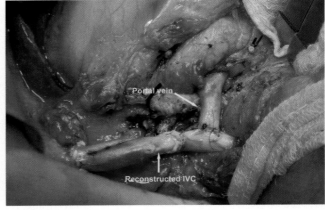

Figure 10-26.

Step 26. Replacement of inadequate native vena cava. Prepare the segment of cadaver donor iliac vein graft, with side branches sutured with vascular suture. Anastomose the interposition graft to the suprahepatic and infrahepatic vena cava (Fig. 10-25).

Step 27. Portacaval shunt created into caval interposition graft. The portacaval shunt can also be created into the interposition graft (Fig. 10-26).

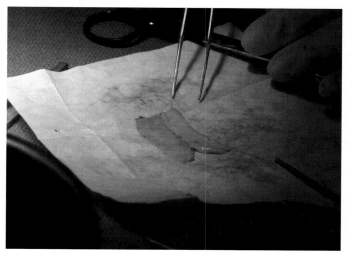

Figure 10-27.

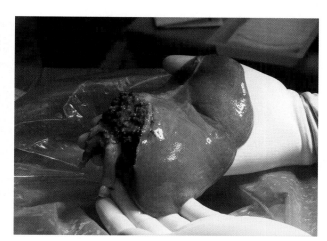

Figure 10-28.

Step 28. Recipient portal vein reconstruction. If the recipient portal vein is unusable, either because it is thrombosed or it is thought to be too small to anastomose to a much larger recipient left portal vein, an interposition graft can be created using a segment of donor saphenous vein. If a single diameter of saphenous vein is too small, the diameter can be doubled by anastomosing two segments together. Each segment is opened along one wall longitudinally, and then they are sewn to each other to create a length with twice the diameter. This composite graft can then be anastomosed to the recipient superior mesenteric vein for the portal venous inflow to the graft. Interposition grafts off the superior mesenteric vein should be tunneled through the transverse mesocolon and anterior to the pancreas (Fig. 10-27).

Step 29. Donor graft prepared. Open the donor left lateral segment packaging. If not already done, weigh and inspect the graft (Fig. 10-28).

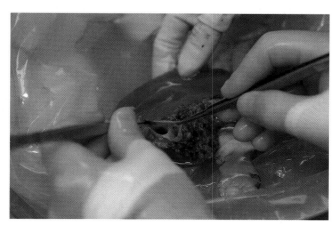

Figure 10-29.

Step 30. Donor hepatic vein. Identify the donor left hepatic vein. In this case, there were two large tributaries that joined to form a large left hepatic vein opening (Fig. 10-29).

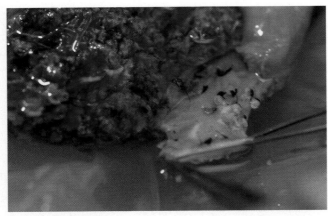

Figure 10-30.

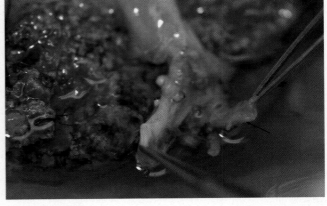

Figure 10-31.

Step 31. Donor portal vein. Inspect the donor left portal vein and place a suture (or a stripe made with a marking pen) to orient the vein (Fig. 10-30).

Step 32. Donor hepatic artery. The forceps on the right side of the photo is on the left hepatic artery (arrow, Fig. 10-31).

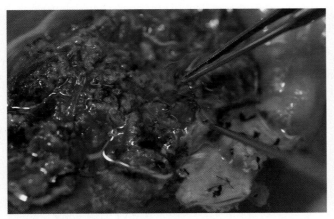

Figure 10-32.

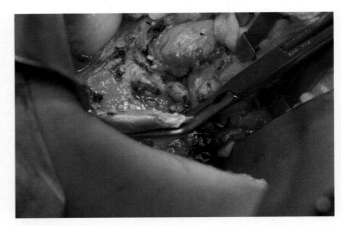

Figure 10-33.

Step 33. Donor bile duct(s). In Figure 10-32, a marking suture has been placed on the bile duct to segments 2 and 3.

Step 34. Hepatic venous anastomosis. The hepatic venous anastomosis is performed first. Join the right, middle, and left hepatic veins of the recipient to form a common opening, after repositioning the vascular clamp. As an alternative, the recipient hepatic veins can be oversewn and the anastomosis to the recipient vena cava can be performed in an end-to-side fashion after a side-biting vascular clamp is applied to the vena cava (as shown in Fig. 10-33).

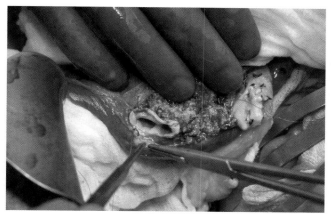

Figure 10-34.

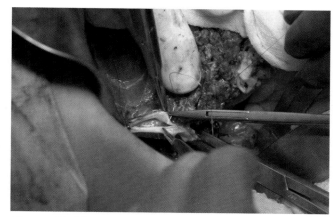

Figure 10-35.

Step 35. Hepatic venous anastomosis (2). Place corner sutures into the left hepatic vein and vena cava (Fig. 10-34).

Step 36. Hepatic venous anastomosis (3). Sew the back wall of the anastomosis from the inside (Fig. 10-35). Disconnect the temporary portacaval shunt. Clamp the portal vein and divide the shunt. Before oversewing the stump of portal vein that is on the vena cava, flush the donor liver with cold Ringer's lactate solution (to remove the residual preservation solution in the graft) through the portal vein. Vent this out the opening in the vena cava, where the portacaval shunt had been created.

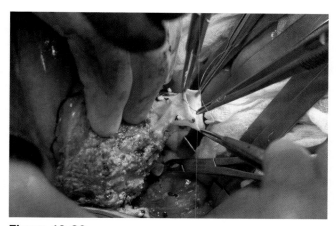

Figure 10-36.

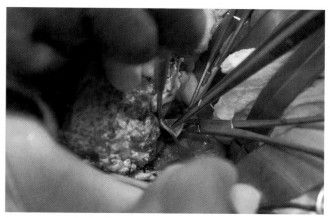

Figure 10-37.

Step 37. Portal vein anastomosis. Perform the portal vein anastomosis. Flush blood out of the recipient portal vein to ensure that no clot has formed. Create an end-to-end anastomosis between the donor left portal vein and the recipient portal vein. Perform a careful orientation of the anastomosis to avoid a twist in either of the vessels. Preplaced marking sutures can aid in orientation (Fig. 10-36).

Step 38. Portal vein anastomosis (2). Perform the anastomosis using a single continuous fine vascular suture. Tie a large "growth factor" knot so that with expansion of the veins, the suture does not constrict the anastomosis. Release the clamps from the vena cava and portal vein, and the graft is revascularized (Fig. 10-37).

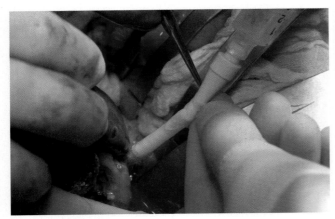

Figure 10-38.

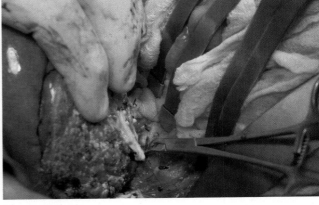

Figure 10-39.

Step 39. Arterial anastomosis. The arterial anastomosis is next performed. Ideally, determine before removing the graft from cold storage whether the recipient artery is of suitable size and length to reach the donor left hepatic artery. If the recipient hepatic artery is not suitable, an interposition graft can be used, either a segment of donor saphenous vein or a segment of cadaveric iliac artery (blood group-compatible). This interposition graft can be placed either onto the supraceliac aorta or the infrarenal aorta if the recipient hepatic artery is not of suitable quality (e.g., too small, dissected) or onto the donor hepatic artery if the recipient artery is of suitable quality but just too short to reach without tension. In Figure 10-38, the graft of cadaver iliac artery was placed after the liver had been revascularized.

Step 40. Arterial interposition graft. Perform the arterial anastomosis between the arterial interposition graft, which has previously been anastomosed to the left hepatic artery, and the recipient's common hepatic artery. Use continuous 8-0 polypropylene suture for the back row and interrupted 8-0 polypropylene suture for the front row. For this anastomosis, use high loupe magnification or an operating microscope (Fig. 10-39).

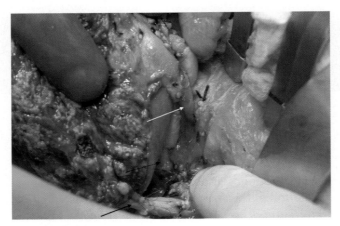

Figure 10-40.

Step 41. Hemostasis achieved. Complete the vascular anastomoses and obtain hemostasis. Inspect the hepatic vein (black arrow), portal vein (white arrow), and hepatic artery (dashed arrow) (Fig. 10-40).

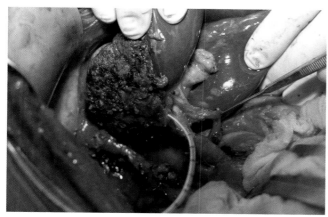
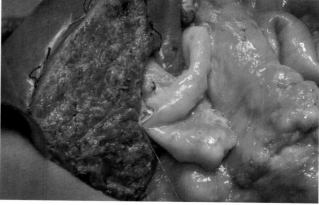

Figure 10-41. **Figure 10-42.**

Step 42. Bile duct inspection. Place an infant feeding tube into the bile duct to segments 2 and 3 to ensure that both have been identified. In this case, the ducts shared a common middle wall. Inspect the bile duct to ensure that the edges are bleeding and appear healthy (Fig. 10-41).

Step 43. Biliary anastomosis. Create the anastomosis to the segment 2 and 3 bile duct with interrupted fine monofilament absorbable suture. Place small infant feeding tubes into both ducts to assist in the anastomosis and prevent catching the back wall. Remove the tubes before the final sutures are placed in the anterior row of the anastomosis. If the ducts to segments 2 and 3 are separate, create two separate hepaticojejunostomies (Fig. 10-42).

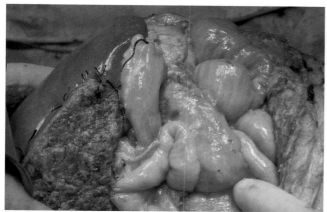
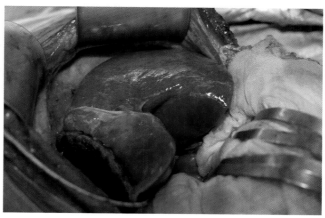

Figure 10-43. **Figure 10-44.**

Step 44. Roux limb secured. Tack the Roux limb to the parenchyma of the liver and to the transverse mesocolon (Fig. 10-43).

Step 45. Liver graft secured. Resuspend the falciform ligament to the diaphragm and peritoneum. Bring a large closed-suction drain through the anterior abdominal wall and lay it near the cut surface of the liver (Fig. 10-44).

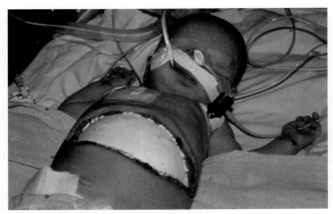

Figure 10-45.

Step 46. Temporary fascial grafts. If the size of the donor graft causes undue abdominal wall or compartment tension during closure, place a fascial patch and downsize it over a period of 7 to 14 days (Fig. 10-45).

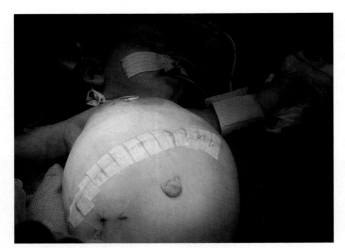

Figure 10-46.

Step 47. Fascial and skin closure. Close the fascia in two layers with absorbable monofilament suture. Close the skin with a subcuticular suture (Fig. 10-46).

Section V

Kidney Transplantation

Chapter 11
Kidney Transplantation

■ **John E. Scarborough, M.D.**
■ **R. Randal Bollinger, M.D., Ph.D.**

Department of Surgery, Duke University Medical Center, Durham, NC

INTRODUCTION

The first long-functioning nonhuman renal transplant was performed in a dog by Emerich Ullmann in 1902. Over the next few decades, several advancements were made in the technical aspects of organ transplantation, including the refinement of vascular anastomoses by Alexis Carrel. The first human kidney transplant procedure was attempted in 1933 in the Ukraine by Voronoy, who transplanted the kidney of a head-injury victim into a patient with acute renal failure from mercuric chloride poisoning. This allograft, and six others performed by Voronoy, failed to produce urine. The first clinically useful human renal allograft was performed by Hufnagel, Hume, and Landsteiner in Boston in 1946. Their procedure involved the transplantation of a human renal allograft to the arm vessels of a patient with transient renal failure. The transplanted kidney functioned temporarily until the recipient's native renal function recovered. The first human renal transplant to achieve long-term function was performed in 1954 by Murray between monozygotic twins. The modern era of immunosuppression was heralded in 1958 by Murray of Boston and Hamburger of Paris, who each performed a series of human kidney allografts using total-body irradiation. Using the modern techniques illustrated in this chapter, currently over 14,000 renal allografts are performed in the United States each year.

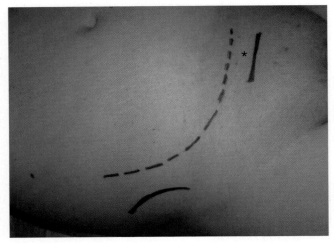

Figure 11-1.

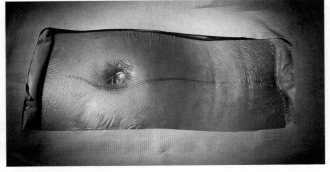

Figure 11-2.

Step 1. Approach. The most common skin incision is a curvilinear one from just above the pubic symphysis (*) to just medial to the anterior superior iliac spine on the side chosen for transplantation. The medial incision, about 2 cm above the symphysis, can be extended across the midline, and the lateral incision, about 2 cm medial to the anterior superior iliac spine, can be extended superiorly in a cephalad direction when circumstances require a larger incision (Fig. 11-1).

Step 2. Approach (2). A lower midline incision is used under special circumstances such as when two aged kidneys are placed in the same recipient, a kidney transplant is performed simultaneously with a pancreas transplant, or when the third or fourth renal transplant is being placed into a patient who has previously had both groins used (Fig. 11-2).

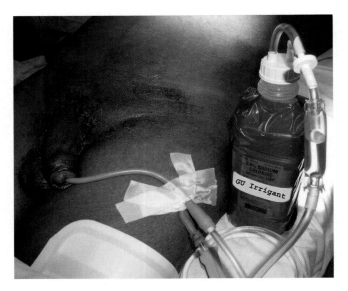

Figure 11-3.

Step 3. Distention of bladder. An 18 Fr Foley catheter is inserted into the urinary bladder, which is then irrigated with an antibiotic solution such as Neosporin GU irrigant. To facilitate distention of the bladder to implant the ureter later in the procedure, cystoscopy tubing may be left attached to the Foley catheter and to a bottle of antibiotic irrigation solution, which can then be elevated and opened in order to irrigate or distend the bladder as necessary (Fig. 11-3).

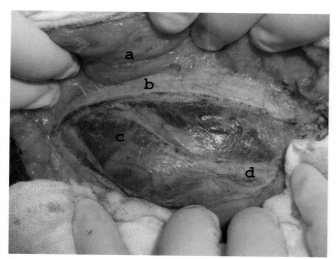

Figure 11-4.

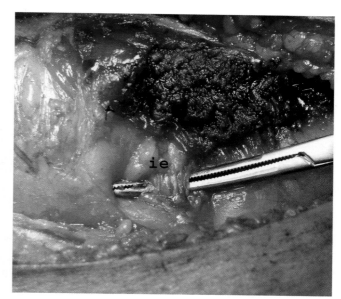

Figure 11-5.

Step 4. Abdominal exposure. Open the layers of the abdominal wall sequentially to expose the underlying peritoneum, which is left intact. The skin, subcutaneous fat (a), Scarpa's fascia, external oblique aponeurosis (b), internal oblique muscle (c), and transversalis fascia (d) are evident in Figure 11-4.

Step 5. Exposure of epigastric vessels. Divide the anterior rectus sheath and rectus muscle to expose the inferior epigastric vessels (ie), which are ligated and divided. The inferior epigastric artery can be used to supply an isolated lower pole renal artery that does not reach easily to the external iliac artery (Fig. 11-5).

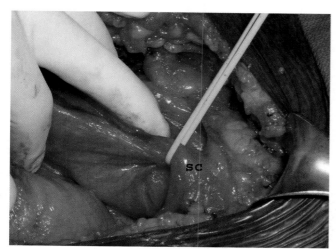

Figure 11-6.

Step 6. Mobilization of spermatic cord. In a male patient, free the spermatic cord (sc) circumferentially and encircle it with a tape, which is used to retract it out of the operative field. If the spermatic cord significantly impairs the subsequent dissection, it may be divided and ligated. Fertility may be affected, but the testicle is usually adequately supplied with blood from the superficial testicular vessels in the floor of the inguinal canal (Fig. 11-6).

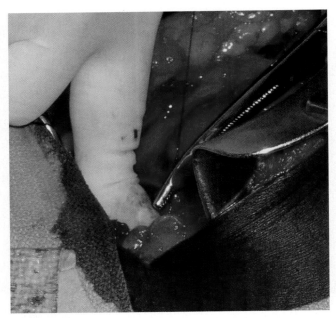

Figure 11-7.

Step 7. Division and ligation of round ligament. In the female patient, identify, double-clamp, divide, and ligate the round ligament to facilitate exposure of the retroperitoneum (Fig. 11-7).

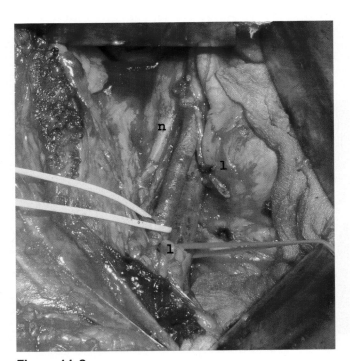

Figure 11-8.

Step 8. Creating pocket for new kidney. Make a retroperitoneal pocket for the new kidney. Carefully preserve the nerves (n) overlying the psoas muscle. No retractor is placed over the femoral nerve in order to avoid compression, which may produce a nerve palsy. Ligate the lymphatics (l) in the areolar tissues surrounding the iliac vessels to avoid postoperative lymphocele (Fig. 11-8).

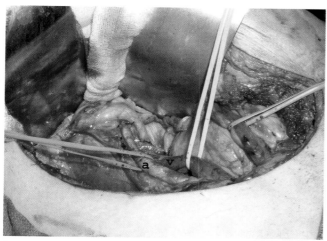

Figure 11-9.

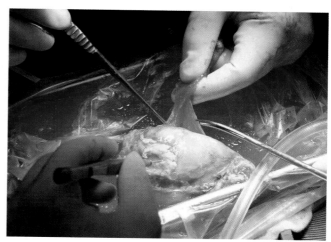

Figure 11-10.

Step 9. Mobilization of external iliac artery and vein. Mobilize the external iliac artery (a) and vein (v) and encircle them with tapes to facilitate traction without injury to the vessels. In infants or small children receiving large kidneys, continue the dissection onto the common iliac artery and aorta to obtain an inflow vessel of adequate size. In such cases, the distal vena cava may also be mobilized through the same approach (Fig. 11-9).

Step 10. Preparation of kidney. Back-table preparation of the kidney includes mobilization of the renal artery and vein, removal of the adrenal gland, and excision of fat between Gerota's fascia and the renal capsule. The capsule of the kidney is left intact. The blood supply to the ureter is preserved by avoiding dissection between the lower pole of the kidney and the transplant ureter (Fig. 11-10).

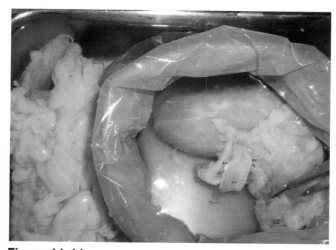

Figure 11-11.

Step 11. Preparation of kidney (2). During preparation, the gonadal vein and adrenal vein are ligated close to the renal vein. Both the artery and the vein are mobilized circumferentially to the level of their first major branches (Fig. 11-11).

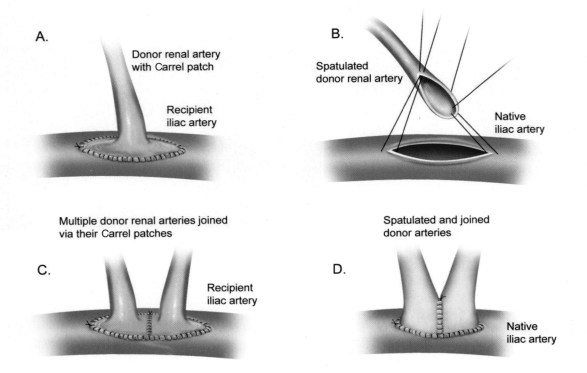

A.
Donor renal artery
with Carrel patch

Recipient
iliac artery

B.
Spatulated
donor renal artery

Native
iliac artery

Multiple donor renal arteries joined
via their Carrel patches

C.
Recipient
iliac artery

Spatulated and joined
donor arteries

D.
Native
iliac artery

Figure 11-12.

Step 12. Preparation of renal artery. Several alternatives for preparation of the renal artery are shown. A Carrel patch of donor aorta (diagram A) provides a useful sewing ring unless there is atherosclerotic narrowing in the donor aorta. Spatulation of the artery (diagram B) will also prevent anastomotic stenosis. In the case of multiple renal arteries, two or more Carrel patches may be sutured together to achieve a single patch for implantation (diagram C). Alternatively, arteries spatulated on their adjacent sides may be anastomosed with fine monofilament suture to achieve a large lumen for anastomosis (diagram D). However, multiple renal arteries may also be anastomosed separately to the iliac system of the recipient (Fig. 11-12).

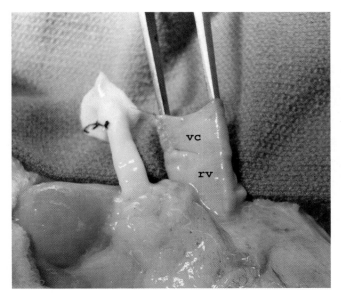

Figure 11-13.

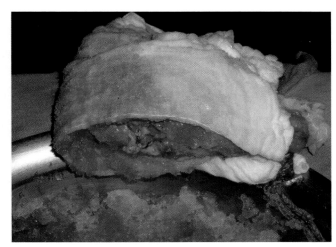

Figure 11-14.

Step 13. Preparation for anastomosis. Whereas the left renal vein is ordinarily sufficiently long to permit primary end-to-side anastomosis to the recipient external iliac vein, extension of the short right renal vein may be necessary. Vena cava harvested with the kidney may be fashioned into a caval conduit (vc) by oversewing one end or by oversewing both ends and using the opening in the opposite side wall where the left renal vein (rv) was excised (Fig. 11-13).

Step 14. Preservation of kidney. To avoid warm ischemia, the kidney is kept packed in ice and wrapped in a sponge or laparotomy pad throughout the time of vascular anastomosis (Fig. 11-14).

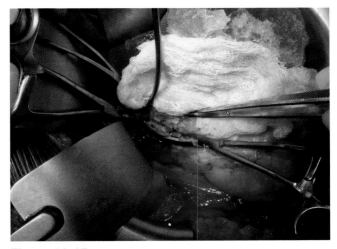

Figure 11-15.

Step 15. Venous anastomosis. The venous anastomosis is performed first. Leave sufficient room for the lower pole of the transplanted kidney to fit between the site chosen for the anastomosis and the inferior wall of the bony pelvis. Clamp the iliac vein above and below the chosen site and make a venotomy by incising the vein or removing a small ellipse of it. Flush the lumen with heparinized saline to eliminate all blood (Fig. 11-15).

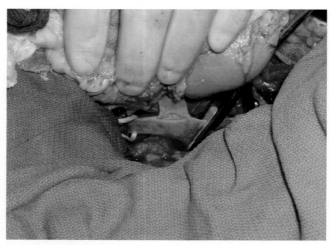

Figure 11-16.

Step 16. Venous anastomosis (2). Sew the venous anastomosis with fine 5-0 or 6-0 monofilament suture. Perform an end-to-side anastomosis by placing stay sutures at the superior and inferior ends of the external iliac venotomy and the corresponding points of the renal vein. The stay sutures are tied down superiorly and inferiorly and then sewn to the midpoint, either by sewing the back wall followed by the front wall, or by sewing one wall from each side of the operating table (Fig. 11-16).

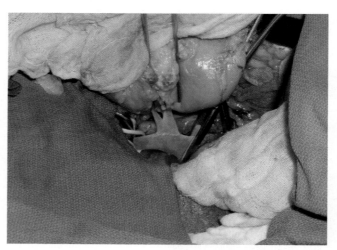

Figure 11-17.

Step 17. Alternatives to venous anastomosis. If the external iliac vein is unsuitable for the venous anastomosis, several alternatives may be considered. Connection to the common iliac vein or vena cava is possible through the same incision. A graft, preferably of autologous internal iliac or saphenous vein, may be used to extend the renal vein length. Allogeneic vessels such as vena cava, iliac vein, iliac artery, or mesenteric vein, when available from the donor of the kidney, make excellent extensions. Conduits made of synthetic material such as polytetrafluoroethylene (PTFE) are less desirable alternatives (Fig. 11-17).

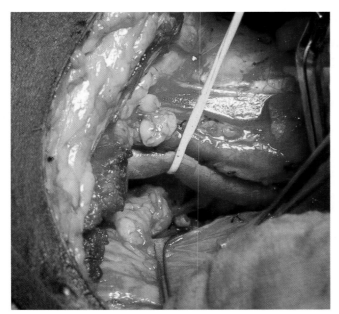

Figure 11-18.

Step 18. Arterial anastomosis. The arterial anastomosis is accomplished after full mobilization of the artery selected to supply the transplant. Mobilization must be adequate to permit proximal and distal control without restricting access to the arteriotomy site. The site of anastomosis must be sufficiently far from the lower pelvic wall to permit easy positioning of the lower pole of the kidney without undue tension on the renal artery. Establish proximal and distal control with vascular clamps and make an arteriotomy. If the recipient artery is thick-walled, a portion of it may be removed with an aortic punch (Fig. 11-18).

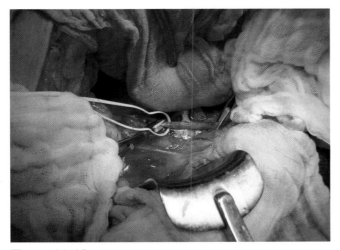

Figure 11-19.

Step 19. Arterial anastomosis (2). Place a double-ended monofilament suture between the renal artery and the external iliac artery posteriorly; continue in both directions until they are joined anteriorly (Fig. 11-19).

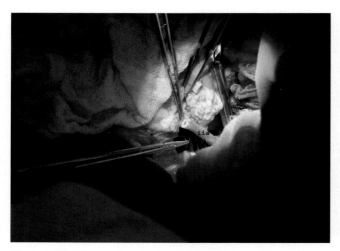

Figure 11-20.

Step 20. Mobilization of internal iliac artery. In recipients with minimal atherosclerosis and well-developed internal iliac arteries, the internal iliac artery may be mobilized and used end-to-end to supply one or more transplant renal arteries. Dissect the internal iliac artery (iia) from the bifurcation of the common iliac artery to the point where it divides into several pelvic branches. Clamp the artery at the iliac artery bifurcation, divide it distally, and flush with heparinized saline. Use a silk tie and suture ligature to secure the distal segment. Rotate the internal iliac artery externally, taking care to avoid kinking of the artery at its origin. Spatulate and suture it end-to-end to the spatulated end of the donor renal artery (Fig. 11-20).

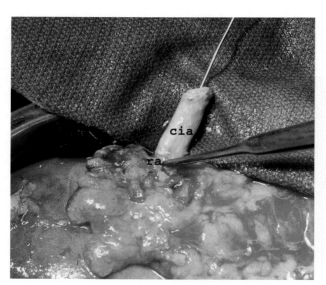

Figure 11-21.

Step 21. Insufficient donor renal artery. If the donor renal artery is of insufficient length for adequate anastomosis, more extensive mobilization of the recipient external iliac artery may be required. Alternatively, common iliac artery (cia) obtained from the cadaver donor or internal iliac artery obtained from the recipient may be attached via an end-to-end anastomosis to the short donor renal artery (ra) to provide more length. Conduits made of synthetic material such as polytetrafluoroethylene (PTFE) or Dacron are additional alternatives (Fig. 11-21).

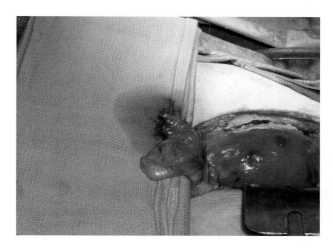

Figure 11-22.

Step 22. Reperfusion of kidney. Prior to reperfusion, the recipient is prepared by administration of immunosuppressive drugs (e.g., steroids, calcineurin inhibitors, monoclonal or polyclonal antibody preparations), diuretics (e.g., mannitol, furosemide), and intravenous fluids to achieve adequate volume loading (i.e., central venous pressure greater than 10 cm H_2O). Remove the venous clamp to demonstrate a patent venous system; then open the renal artery to reperfuse the kidney with warm, oxygenated blood. Any additional sutures required for hemostasis are taken before the kidney is rewarmed. In a patient with adequate filling pressure and normal arterial pressure, the transplanted kidney rapidly gains turgor, becomes pink, and begins to produce urine. Failure in any of these respects warrants immediate investigation to rule out obstruction from thrombus, embolus, stenosis, or hypotension (Fig. 11-22).

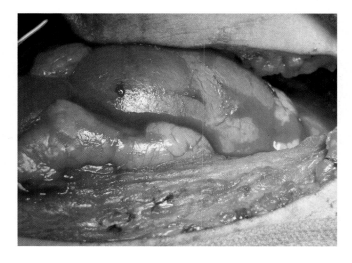

Figure 11-23.

Step 23. Positioning of kidney. Position the kidney in the fossa created by the iliac crest. By placing the kidney into the side opposite from its origin, the posterior surface of the kidney, the ureter, and the renal pelvis are now anterior. The renal vein has a shorter distance to traverse in order to reach the external iliac vein. The renal artery lies anterior to the vein and reaches easily to the external iliac, internal iliac, or common iliac artery site chosen for the arterial anastomosis (Fig. 11-23).

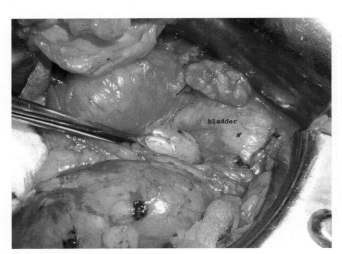

Figure 11-24.

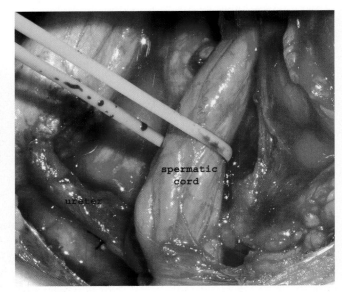

Figure 11-25.

Step 24. Distention of bladder. Distend the urinary bladder with an antibiotic irrigation solution through the reservoir and cystoscopy tubing attached to the Foley catheter. Identify the peritoneal reflection on the anterior surface of the bladder and either avoid it or mobilize it away from the site of the ureteral anastomosis (Fig. 11-24).

Step 25. Positioning of transplant ureter. Bring the transplant ureter posterior to the spermatic cord to avoid kinking and urinary obstruction (Fig. 11-25).

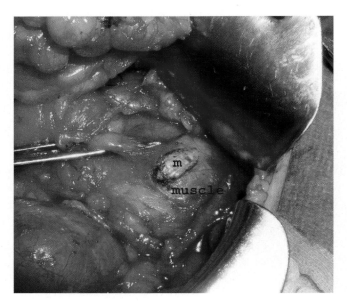

Figure 11-26.

Step 26. Creation of antireflux tunnel. Make an incision through the serosal and muscular layers of the bladder wall over a distance of 3 cm in the direction of the transplant ureter. The mucosa (m) of the fluid-filled bladder is dark in contrast to the overlying pale muscle. Clear the mucosa for the length of the incision and laterally for a distance of 5 mm on each side to permit creation of an antireflux tunnel (Fig. 11-26).

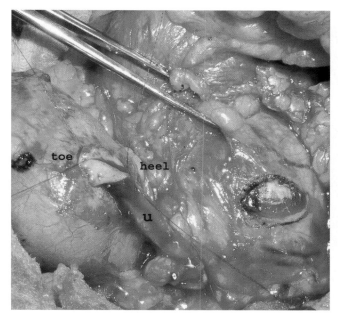

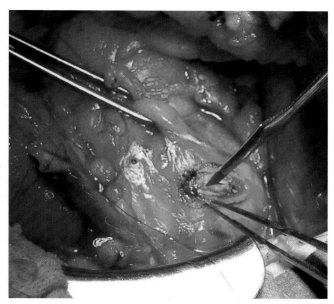

Figure 11-27.   **Figure 11-28.**

Step 27. Spatulate ureter. Cut the transplant ureter to length and spatulate it. Preplace anchor sutures of 6-0 absorbable suture material in the toe and heel of the spatulated ureter (u) (Fig. 11-27).

Step 28. Identification of mucosal edges. Incise the bladder and place the two anchor sutures through the bladder wall while the irrigant is flowing through the mucosal incision to facilitate easy identification of the mucosal edges and proper placement of the fixation structures (Fig. 11-28).

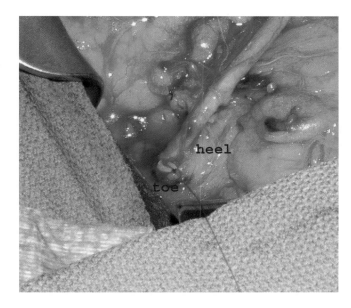

Figure 11-29.

Step 29. Anastomosis between ureter and bladder. Place the medial suture from the toe of the ureter through all layers of the bladder wall to anchor the ureter; in contrast, place the heel suture through mucosa only. Perform the anastomosis between the ureter and the bladder mucosa with running 6-0 absorbable suture (Fig. 11-29).

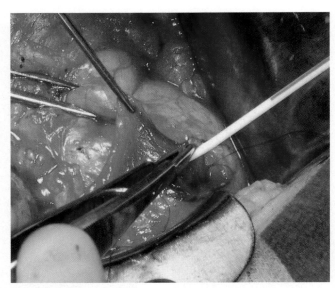

Figure 11-30.

Step 30. Stenting transplanted kidney. A 6 Fr double-J ureteral stent, either 12 or 16 cm long depending on the length of the transplant ureter, may be placed via the ureteral orifice into the collecting system of the transplanted kidney, with the other end into the urinary bladder (Fig. 11-30).

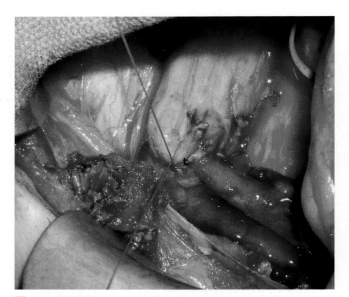

Figure 11-31.

Step 31. Creating antireflux tunnel. Create the antireflux tunnel (t) by closing the bladder muscle over the top of the implanted ureter using interrupted 4-0 absorbable suture (Fig. 11-31).

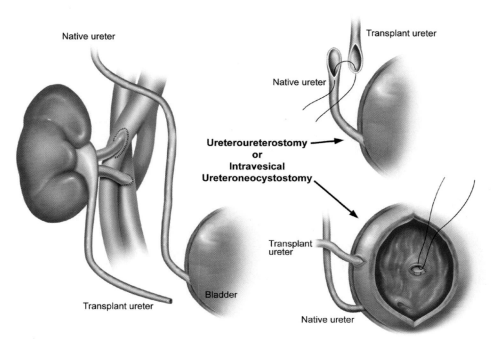

Figure 11-32.

Step 32. Attaching transplanted ureter. Two alternative methods of attaching the transplant ureter (left diagram) to the recipient urinary system are shown. The ureteroureterostomy (upper right diagram) is performed with interrupted absorbable sutures between the spatulated end of the transplant ureter and the remnant of the recipient's native ureter after removal of the kidney on that side. A double-J stent may be placed through the ureters between the renal pelvis of the transplant and the bladder of the recipient. An intravesical method of ureteroneocystostomy (lower right diagram) is performed by opening the bladder with an anterior, lateral incision, incising the bladder mucosa from inside, and drawing the transplant ureter through a 2.5-cm submucosal tunnel. The ureter is sutured to the mucosa of the bladder with interrupted 4-0 sutures, an optional ureteral stent is placed, and the bladder wall incision is closed with running absorbable sutures for the mucosal, the muscular, and the serosal layers. Regardless of the type of ureteral attachment, some redundancy of the ureter is left outside the bladder to permit easy positioning of the kidney and to allow for some movement (Fig. 11-32).

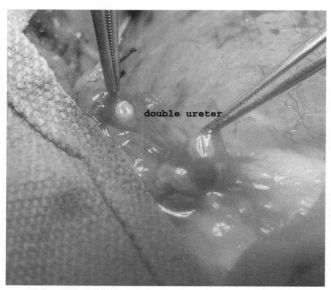

Figure 11-33.

Step 33. Management of double ureter. Occasionally the donor kidney has a double ureter. These cases may be managed by spatulating the two ureters, suturing them together, and then implanting them as a single unit (Fig. 11-33). However, urinary leaks are less likely to occur if each ureter is implanted separately, either by using the extravesical (Figs. 11-23 to 11-30) technique twice or by using the intravesical (Fig. 11-31) technique with separate mucosal openings and attachments for each ureter.

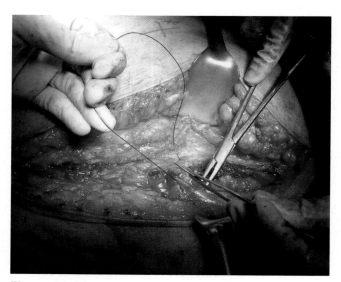

Figure 11-34.

Step 34. Closure. Close the abdominal wound using the external oblique and anterior rectus sheath. The internal oblique and rectus muscles may be excluded to avoid injury to the underlying colon. Scarpa's fascia may be closed with a running, absorbable suture. Close the skin with staples (Fig. 11-34).

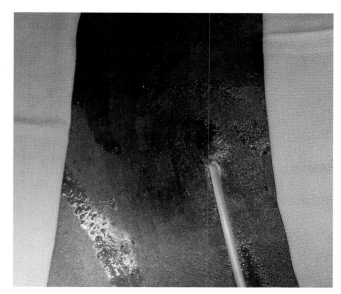

Figure 11-35.

Step 35. Tenckhoff catheter removal. If prompt, brisk urine production from the new transplant is evident, patients with peritoneal dialysis access catheters may have them removed during the same anesthesia (Fig. 11-35).

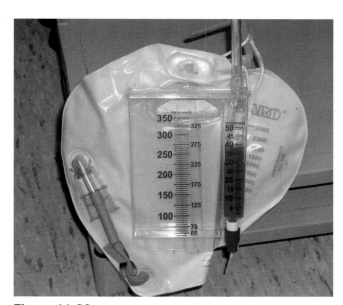

Figure 11-36.

Step 36. Dressing and extubation. Place a sterile dressing over the abdominal wound and the old Tenckhoff catheter site as applicable. Attach a urometer to the Foley catheter. The patient is then awakened and extubated for transport to a recovery unit (Fig. 11-36).

EN BLOC TRANSPLANTATION

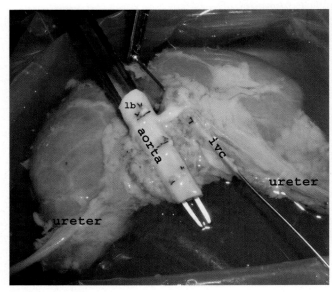

Figure 11-37.

Step 1. En bloc transplantation. Pediatric kidneys when implanted singly have a demonstrably lower rate of function, so both kidneys from young donors are often transplanted en bloc. Prepare the vena cava (ivc) of the donor by ligating all its nonrenal branches. Similarly ligate the lumbar branches (lb) of the donor aorta. Suture shut the proximal ends of the donor vena cava and aorta; an aortic patch is often used for the arterial closure (Fig. 11-37).

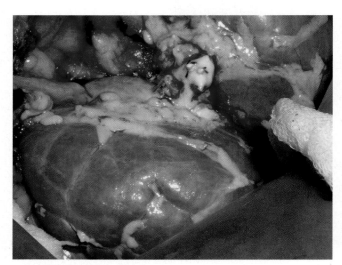

Figure 11-38.

Step 2. En bloc transplantation (2). Suture the vena cava and aorta to the recipient external iliac vein and artery, respectively. Implant the ureters separately into the bladder over small double-J stents using the techniques described previously (Fig. 11-38).

Laparoscopic Living-Donor Nephrectomy

■ **Lloyd E. Ratner, M.D.**

Department of Surgery, Thomas Jefferson University Hospital, Philadelphia, PA

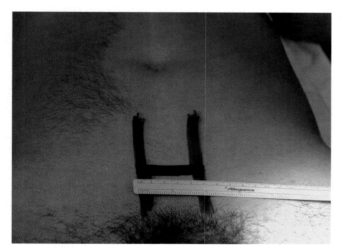

Figure 12-1.

Step 1. Preparation. After general anesthesia has been induced, and with the patient in the supine position, mark a 5-cm Pfannenstiel incision two fingerbreadths superior to the pubis. A Foley catheter is inserted and intermittent compression stockings are placed on the lower extremities (Fig. 12-1).

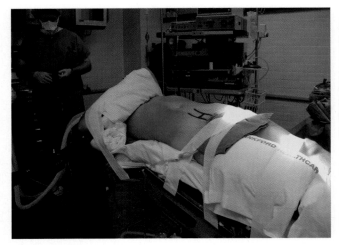

Figure 12-2.

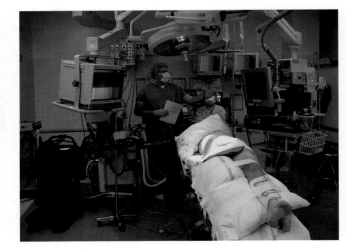

Figure 12-3.

Step 2. Patient positioning. The patient is turned to a modified lateral decubitus position. The hips are rolled posteriorly to allow easier access to the Pfannenstiel incision. The arms are crossed across the chest and the patient is taped securely to the operating table. The table is then placed in the full flex position. A robotic arm is attached to the right side of the table. Monitors are positioned adjacent to the left and right shoulders (Figs. 12-2 and 12-3).

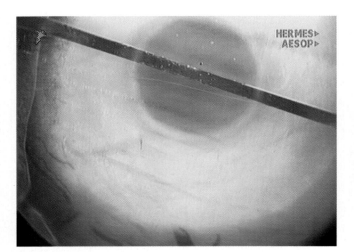

Figure 12-4.

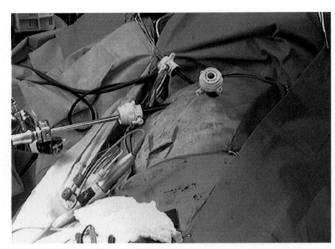

Figure 12-5.

Step 3. Insufflation of abdomen. Insert a Veress needle in the lower abdomen (ipsilateral to the kidney to be removed) along the lateral border of the rectus abdominis muscle. Insufflate the abdomen with carbon dioxide to a pressure of 15 mm Hg. Remove the Veress needle, and at the same position insert a 12-mm port under laparoscopic vision using a visual obturator (Fig. 12-4).

Step 4. Insertion of ports. Insert a 5-mm port three fingerbreadths inferior to the xiphoid process. Insert a second 12-mm port at the umbilicus. Place both of these ports under laparoscopic vision. Suture all ports in place at the skin to prevent accidental dislodgement. For right laparoscopic donor nephrectomies, place two subxiphoid ports, one and four fingerbreadths inferior to the xiphoid. The more superior port is used to retract the right lobe of the liver anteriorly (Fig. 12-5).

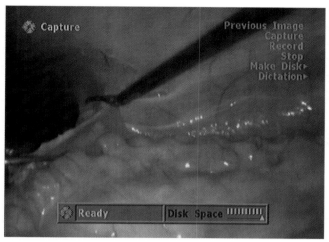

Figure 12-6.

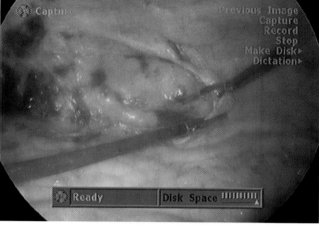

Figure 12-7.

Step 5. Dissection. Begin the dissection by dividing the lateral peritoneal reflection from the splenic flexure to the pelvic inlet. Avoid dissecting posterior to the kidney at this point, so that the posterolateral renal attachments remain intact until after the hilar dissection is complete. On the right side, dissection proceeds from the hepatic flexure to the cecum (Figs. 12-6 and 12-7).

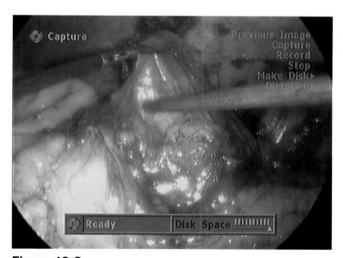

Figure 12-8.

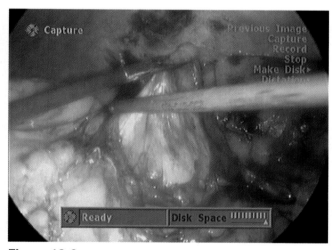

Figure 12-9.

Step 6. Dissection of avascular plane. Continue the dissection in the avascular plane between the descending colonic mesentery anteromedially and Gerota's fascia posterolaterally. Most of this dissection can be performed bluntly. Avoid making a rent in the colonic mesentery (Figs. 12-8 and 12-9).

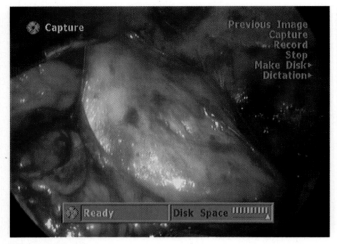

Figure 12-10.

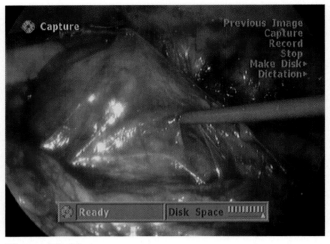

Figure 12-11.

Step 7. Dissection of avascular plane (2). Continue the dissection in this plane until you identify the gonadal vein (Fig. 12-10).

Step 8. Elevation of gonadal vein and ureter. Elevate the gonadal vein, the ureter, and the lower pole of the kidney anterolaterally off the psoas muscle posteriorly (Fig. 12-11).

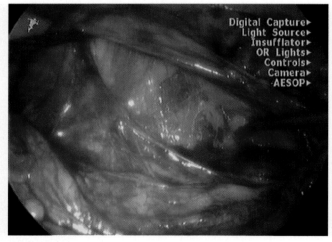

Figure 12-12.

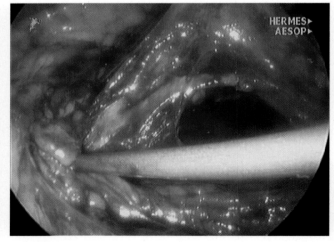

Figure 12-13.

Step 9. Dissection of ureter and gonadal vein. Continue the dissection of the ureter and gonadal vein inferiorly to the level of the iliac vessels (Fig. 12-12).

Step 10. Identification of renal vein. Follow the gonadal vein superiorly until you identify the renal vein (Fig. 12-13).

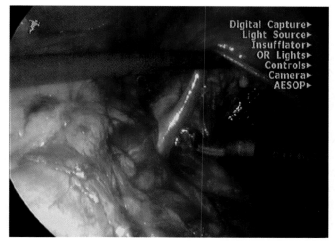

Figure 12-14.

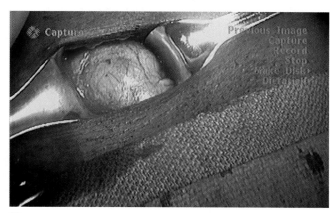

Figure 12-15.

Step 11. Identification of lumbar vein. Continue the dissection along the inferior border of the renal vein, with identification of a lumbar vein off the posterior aspect of the left renal vein (Fig. 12-14).

Step 12. Pfannenstiel incision. Make a 5-cm Pfannenstiel incision two finger-breadths superior to the pubis. Incise the linea alba vertically. Retract the rectus abdominis muscles laterally; the peritoneum pouts out due to the pneumoperitoneum (Fig. 12-15).

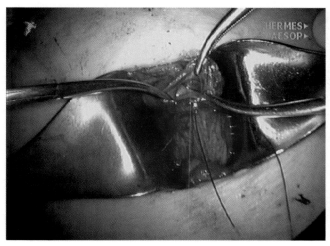
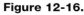

Figure 12-16.

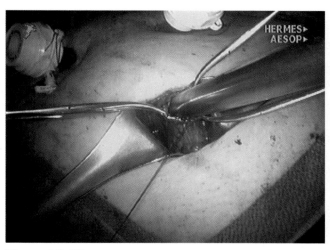

Figure 12-17.

Step 13. Purse-string suture. Place a purse-string suture within the peritoneum through the Pfannenstiel incision. Make a small incision into the peritoneum within the confines of the purse-string (Fig. 12-16).

Step 14. Insertion of Endocatch bag. Insert a 15-mm Endocatch bag through this incision. Securely cinch down the purse-string to maintain the pneumoperitoneum (Fig. 12-17).

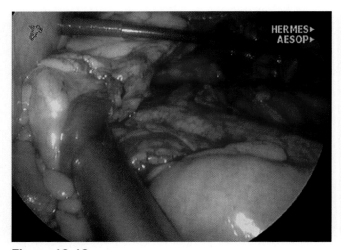

Figure 12-18.

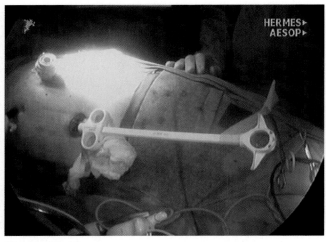

Figure 12-19.

Step 15. **Medial retraction of colon and duodenum.** Use the metal sleeve of the Endocatch bag as a retractor for medial retraction of the colon and duodenum (Fig. 12-18).

Step 16. **Endocatch bag as retractor.** A Penrose drain attached to the drapes enables the Endocatch bag to be used as a self-retaining retractor (Fig. 12-19).

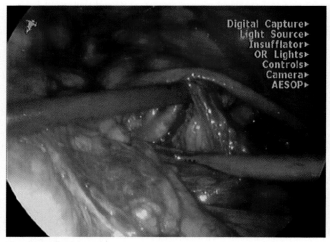

Figure 12-20.

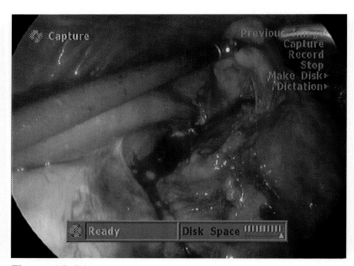

Figure 12-21.

Step 17. **Division of lymphatics and neural tissue.** Divide the lymphatics and neural tissue surrounding and crossing the left renal artery (Fig. 12-20).

Step 18. **Mobilization of upper pole.** Incise Gerota's fascia overlying the anterior surface of the upper pole of the kidney to begin mobilizing the upper pole (Fig. 12-21).

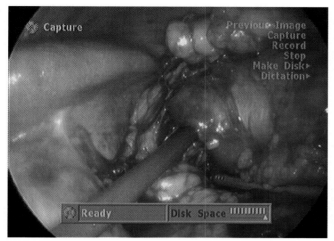

Figure 12-22.

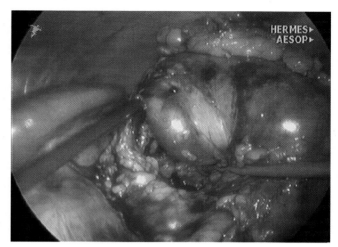

Figure 12-23.

Step 19. Mobilization of upper pole (2). Identify the medial aspect of the upper pole of the kidney by lateral and anterior rotation of the kidney with the instrument passed through the left lower quadrant port. This is frequently the most difficult part of the operation (Fig. 12-22).

Step 20. Mobilization of upper pole (3). Elevate the upper pole of the kidney, with division of its medial and posterior attachments (Fig. 12-23).

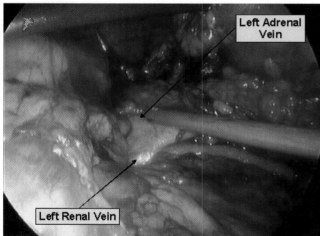

Figure 12-24.

Figure 12-25.

Step 21. Vascular dissection. Continue the dissection medially along the superior aspect of the left renal vein (Fig. 12-24).

Step 22. Identification of left adrenal vein. Identify the left adrenal vein. Usually it enters the renal vein medial to the gonadal vein (Fig. 12-25).

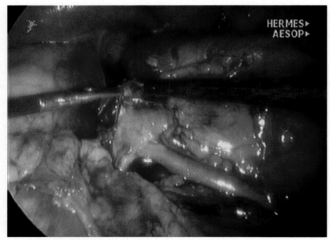

Figure 12-26.

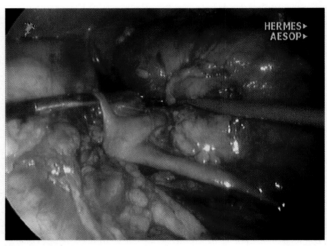

Figure 12-27.

Step 23. Division of left adrenal vein. Dissect, clip, and divide the left adrenal vein (Figs. 12-26 and 12-27).

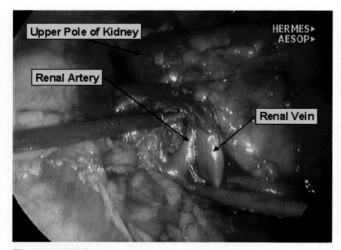

Figure 12-28.

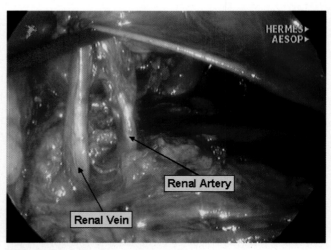

Figure 12-29.

Step 24. Identification of left renal artery. Reflect the left renal vein inferiorly to allow identification of the superior aspect of the left renal artery (Fig. 12-28).

Step 25. Vascular dissection. After dividing the attachments between the superior border of the left renal artery and the left adrenal gland, the vascular dissection is essentially complete (Fig. 12-29).

Chapter 12: Laparoscopic Living-Donor Nephrectomy

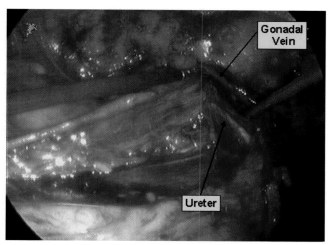

Figure 12-30.

Step 26. Dissection of left gonadal vein and ureter. Attention is turned to the left gonadal vein and ureter, which are dissected inferiorly along the medial aspect of the left gonadal vein to avoid devascularizing the allograft ureter. Divide the gonadal vein at the point where the vein crosses the left ureter (Fig. 12-30).

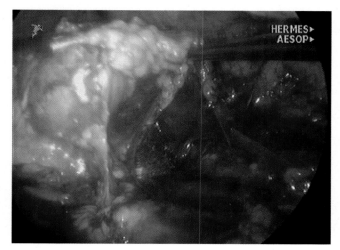

Figure 12-31.

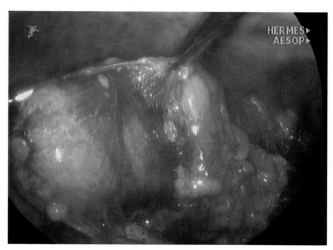

Figure 12-32.

Step 27. Division of lateral and posterior attachments. Mobilize the remainder of the kidney by dividing the lateral and posterior attachments (Figs. 12-31 and 12-32).

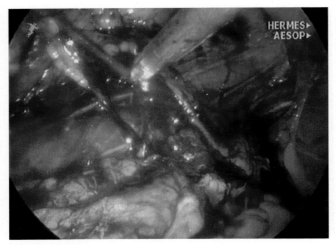

Figure 12-33.

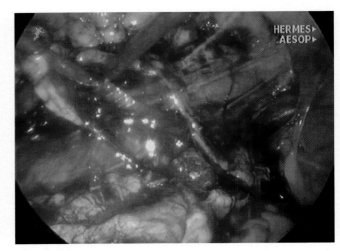

Figure 12-34.

Step 28. Division of distal ureter. Clip and divide the distal ureter proximal to the clips at the point where it crosses the iliac vessels (Figs. 12-33 and 12-34).

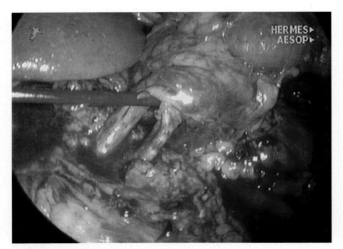

Figure 12-35.

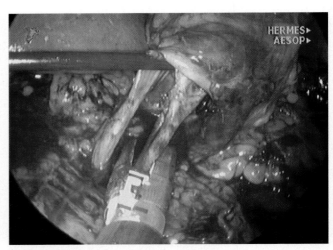

Figure 12-36.

Step 29. Elevation of kidney. Switch the scope from the umbilical to the left lower quadrant port. Pass the left-hand instrument from the subxiphoid port between the renal artery and vein to elevate the kidney anterolaterally in preparation for division of the renal artery. This maneuver maximizes the length of renal artery that will be obtained (Fig. 12-35).

Step 30. Division of renal artery. Pass an Endo-GIA stapler through the umbilical port and use it to divide the renal artery at its origin at the aorta (Fig. 12-36).

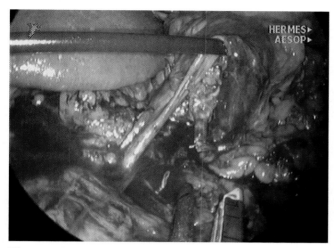

Figure 12-37.

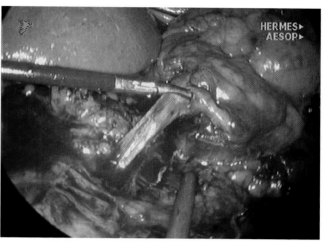

Figure 12-38.

Step 31. Examination of arterial stump. Survey the arterial stump for bleeding, and clip it if necessary (Fig. 12-37).

Step 32. Retraction of renal vein. Grasp the renal vein with an atraumatic forceps and retract it laterally so that maximal length can be obtained. Identify the adrenal vein stump (Fig. 12-38).

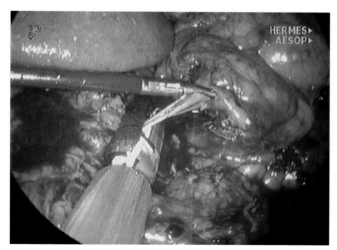

Figure 12-39.

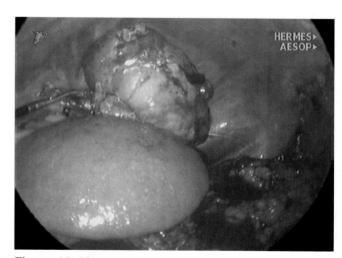

Figure 12-40.

Step 33. Division of left renal vein. Once again pass the Endo-GIA stapler through the umbilical port and use it to divide the left renal vein medial to the adrenal vein stump (Fig. 12-39).

Step 34. Positioning of kidney. After dividing the renal vasculature, flip the kidney up over the spleen (Fig. 12-40).

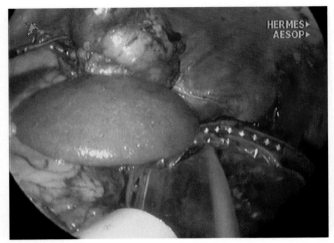

Figure 12-41.

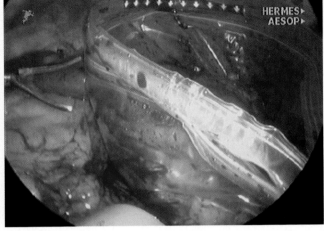

Figure 12-42.

Step 35. Endocatch deployment. Deploy the Endocatch bag within the renal bed (Fig. 12-41).

Step 36. Ensnarement of kidney. Flip the kidney down into the Endocatch bag from its position above the spleen (Fig. 12-42).

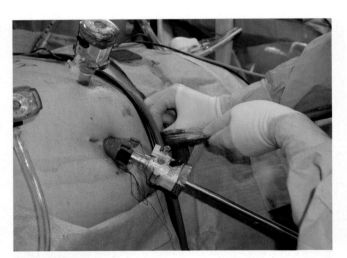

Figure 12-43.

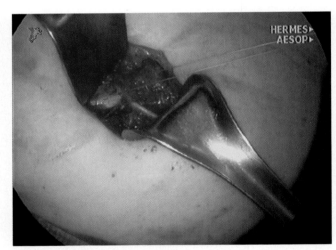

Figure 12-44.

Step 37. Kidney extraction. Extract the kidney from the Pfannenstiel incision within the Endocatch bag (Fig. 12-43).

Step 38. Reapproximation of linea alba. Reapproximate the linea alba through the Pfannenstiel incision with figure-of-eight absorbable sutures. Initially leave one suture untied so that an additional port can be placed, in case a retractor is necessary when assessing the abdomen for hemostasis (Fig. 12-44).

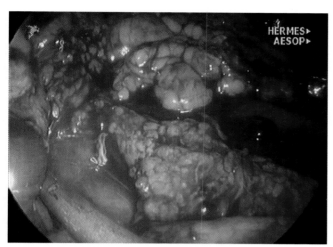

Figure 12-45.

Step 39. Examination of abdomen. Once pneumoperitoneum is re-established, survey the abdomen for hemostasis. Identify the renal arterial stump and the stump of the renal vein (Fig. 12-45).

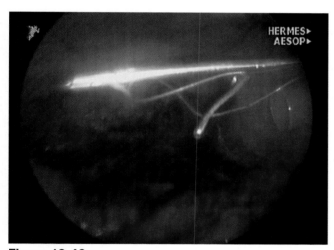

Figure 12-46.

Step 40. Closure. Place figure-of-eight absorbable sutures around the 12-mm port sites under laparoscopic vision using a needle closure device. Then remove the ports and reapproximate the skin incisions (Fig. 12-46).

Section VI

Pancreas Transplantation

Chapter 13
Pancreas Transplantation

■ **Donald C. Dafoe, M.D.**
■ **Lloyd E. Ratner, M.D.**

Department of Surgery, Thomas Jefferson University Hospital, Philadelphia, PA

INTRODUCTION

The modern era of diabetes management began in 1922 with the first clinical use of insulin. Before then, most insulinopenic diabetics had little hope of surviving for more than a few years. Since then, the death rate among diabetics due to coma has been reduced to less than 1%. It is a miracle of modern medicine that most diabetics can now expect a relatively normal lifespan. However, despite the recent advances in the treatment of diabetes, patients still experience a suboptimal quality of life because of dietary restrictions, as well as the need for glucose monitoring and insulin injections. Those who cannot achieve glycemic stability despite their best efforts must live with possibly fatal hypoglycemic reactions or accept the consequences of chronic hyperglycemia, including retinopathy, nephropathy, neuropathy, and accelerated atherosclerosis. Many of these unfortunate patients resign themselves to progressive mixtures of dialysis, blindness, lower extremity pain and numbness, nausea, vomiting, diarrhea, constipation, stroke, heart attack, and amputation. Pancreas transplantation can vastly improve the diabetic's quality of life by normalizing the blood sugar, thereby reducing the risk of secondary complication progression.

Step 1. Positioning. The recipient of the pancreas transplant is positioned supine on the operating table. After general endotracheal anesthesia is induced, a urinary bladder catheter and a central venous line are placed. A self-retaining retractor, such as a Bookwalter or Thompson, is used.

Step 2. Pancreas allograft preparation. Preparation of the pancreas allograft is done in an iced basin. Usually, the whole organ pancreas allograft is procured in the setting of a multi-organ recovery from a deceased donor. Ligate and divide the gas-

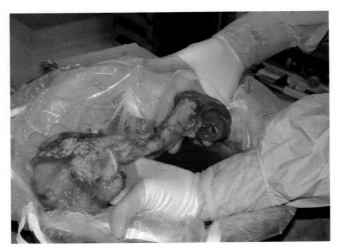

Figure 13-1.

troduodenal artery. The celiac axis accompanies the liver allograft. Ligate the splenic artery on the celiac side; the end on the pancreas side is left open. Transect the superior mesenteric artery (SMA) flush with the aorta in the donor. (A Carrel patch of donor aorta is not necessary and might compromise the lumina of the renal arteries in the donor.) The whole organ pancreas allograft includes a segment of donor duodenum stapled distal to the pylorus and extending beyond the mesenteric vessels. The spleen is attached. The portal vein is divided in the donor, giving the majority of the length to the liver allograft. Typically, 1 to 3 cm of portal vein is left on the pancreas. The extensive branching of the SMA and superior mesenteric vein (SMV) just beyond the uncinate notch of the pancreas graft is stapled en masse with a vascular stapler or oversewn in the donor after in situ flushing (Fig. 13-1).

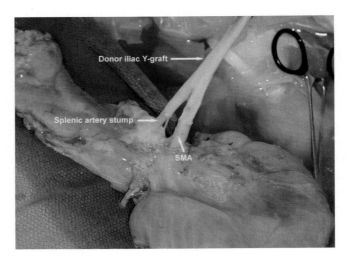

Figure 13-2.

Step 3. Pancreas allograft preparation (2). Reconstruct the arterial blood supply to the pancreas using a donor iliac Y-graft consisting of the common iliac artery with its bifurcation into the internal and external iliac arteries. Sew the larger-diameter internal iliac artery of the Y-graft end-to-end onto the SMA of the pancreas; the external iliac artery of the donor Y-graft is compatible in size with the splenic artery of the pancreas. Perform these anastomoses with 6-0 polypropylene (Fig. 13-2).

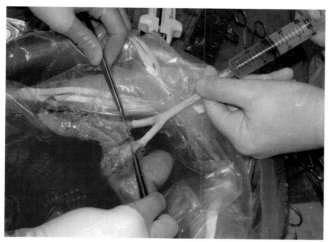

Figure 13-3.

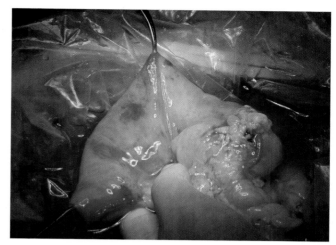

Figure 13-4.

Step 4. Pancreas allograft preparation (3). Perfuse the pancreas with cold solution to check for leaks at the anastomoses or small branches (Fig. 13-3).

Step 5. Pancreas allograft preparation (4). The procurement team usually leaves the duodenum long (Fig. 13-4).

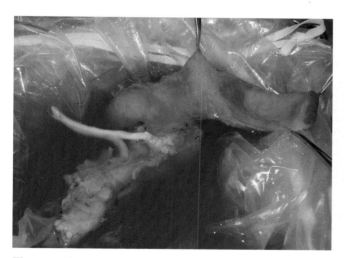

Figure 13-5.

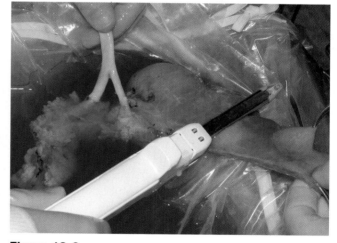

Figure 13-6.

Step 6. Pancreas allograft preparation (5). Starting inferiorly, meticulously clamp the anterior and posterior arcades from the pancreaticoduodenal vessels with a series of mosquito clamps. Divide them. Ligate the pedicles with silk on the pancreas side. As you reach the end of the duodenal segment, also place clamps and ties on the duodenal side. Shorten the graft duodenum to 8 to 10 cm (Fig. 13-5).

Step 7. Pancreas allograft preparation (6). Divide the excess duodenum with a stapling device (Fig. 13-6).

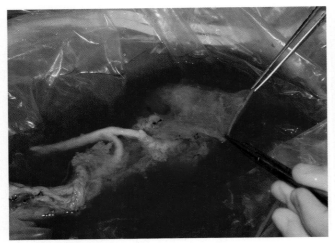

Figure 13-7.

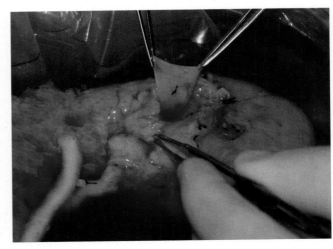

Figure 13-8.

Step 8. Pancreas allograft preparation (7). There is no need to oversew the ends of the duodenal segment, both proximal and distal (Fig. 13-7).

Step 9. Pancreas allograft preparation (8). The portal vein may appear short at first; most of the portal vein goes with the liver graft. In most cases, this is not a problem. In fact, lengthening the portal vein with a segment of donor iliac vein is not recommended as it is thought to be associated with an increased incidence of graft thrombosis. The portal vein length is gained by dissecting it free from surrounding tissues. Ligate larger venous branches and suture small diaphanous branches with a 6-0 polypropylene figure-of-eight stitch (Fig. 13-8).

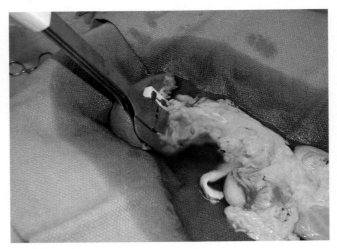

Figure 13-9.

Step 10. Pancreas allograft preparation (9). Perform a graft splenectomy using a vascular stapler. Some surgeons prefer to leave the spleen on the pancreas to use as a handle, thus avoiding graft manipulation. Some surgeons regard the intact spleen as a helpful indicator of venous torsion or obstruction as evidenced by splenic swelling. The staple line often requires a few reinforcing figure-of-eight sutures for hemostasis upon release of the vascular clamps and reperfusion (Fig. 13-9).

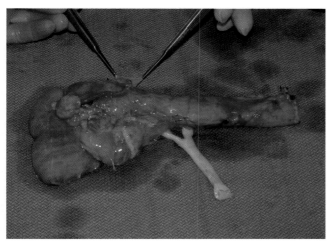

Figure 13-10.

Step 11. Pancreas allograft preparation (10). The pancreaticoduodenal graft is prepared and ready to be brought up into the field for implantation. Figure 13-10 is an anterior view showing the Y-graft, the duodenal segment, and the portal vein.

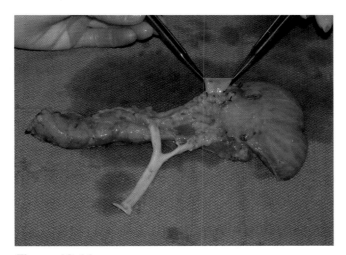

Figure 13-11.

Step 12. Pancreas allograft preparation (11). Figure 13-11 shows a posterior view of the prepared graft. Reflush the pancreas graft with preservation solution through the Y-graft. This practice appears to protect against graft thrombosis. With the reflush, the portal vein effluent clears. Ideally, while the back-basin graft preparation is underway, another team proceeds with the recipient operation.

Step 13. Recipient operation. Make a midline incision from 12 cm above the umbilicus down to the symphysis pubis. Carry the incision through the linea alba. Explore the abdomen for tumor, infection, or other findings that might preclude transplantation. Palpate the gallbladder for stones; we believe that the finding of gallstones is an indication for incidental cholecystectomy after the pancreas trans-

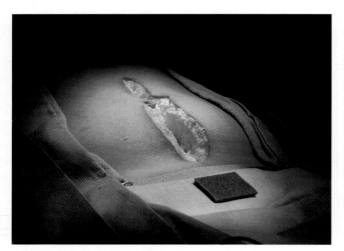

Figure 13-12.

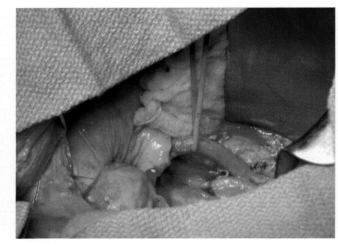

Figure 13-13.

plant is completed. Position a nasogastric tube in the stomach. Perform a Cattell maneuver by scoring the line of Toldt lateral to the right colon, then mobilizing the cecum and terminal ileum off the retroperitoneum by dividing the avascular root of the mesentery. (These maneuvers are similar to those performed for organ procurement.) The retroperitoneum is thus exposed. Place the patient in moderate Trendelenburg position to shift the intestines out of the pelvis, thereby improving exposure. Pack the intestines superiorly and laterally to the left (Fig. 13-12).

Step 14. Isolation of external iliac artery and vein. Isolate the external iliac artery and vein for a distance of 8 to 10 cm, similar to kidney transplant exposure. Because the surgery is intraperitoneal, ligating and dividing lymphatics overlying the vessels is not necessary (Fig. 13-13).

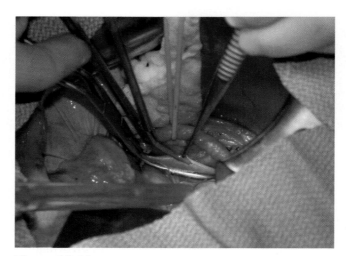

Figure 13-14.

Step 15. Clamping the vessels. Before clamping the recipient vessels, we prefer to anticoagulate therapeutically with heparin. Place a Satinsky or other vascular clamp on the recipient external iliac vein. Make a venotomy with a #11 blade and a Potts scissors to match the size of the graft portal vein, typically about 20 to 24 mm (Fig. 13-14).

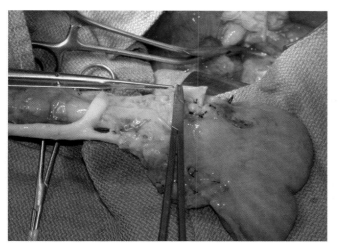

Figure 13-15.

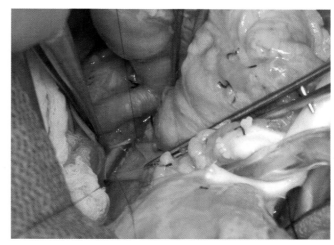

Figure 13-16.

Step 16. Portal vein anastomosis. Bring the pancreas up to the field. Orient it parallel to the recipient vessels, with the graft duodenum facing superiorly. Direct the tail of the pancreas toward the pelvis. Complete the end-to-side venous anastomosis using 5-0 polypropylene (Fig. 13-15).

Step 17. Portal vein anastomosis (2) (Fig. 13-16).

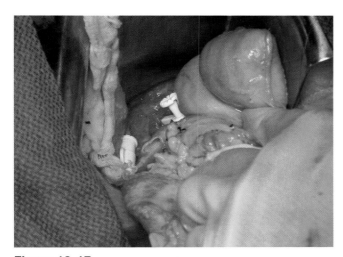

Figure 13-17.

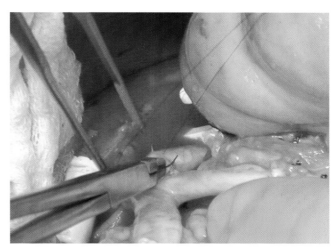

Figure 13-18.

Step 18. Arterial anastomosis. The external iliac artery is controlled with bulldogs in this example. Make an anterior arteriotomy using a #11 blade. Enlarge and round this with a 4-mm aortic punch, fired two or three times (Fig. 13-17).

Step 19. Arterial anastomosis (2). Shorten the common iliac artery of the Y-graft and sew it to the side of the external iliac artery using 6-0 polypropylene. The sew-in time (the time interval from removal of the pancreas graft from ice to reperfusion with oxygenated blood) is typically about 30 minutes (Fig. 13-18). Remove the clamps at the completion of the anastomoses. There are often several bleeding points due to the en bloc procurement of the pancreas, and these are rapidly controlled. Warn the anesthesiologist about the possible need for volume replacement.

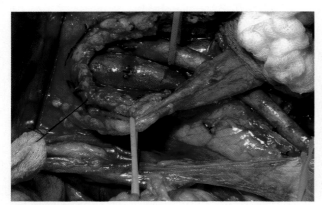

Figure 13-19.

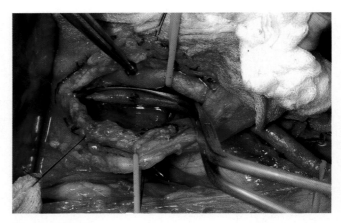

Figure 13-20.

Step 20. Alternative anastomotic site. There are alternate sites for transplantation for the pancreas other than the external iliac vessels. The inferior vena cava (IVC) just above the confluence of the iliac veins is an attractive site for venous drainage (Fig. 13-19).

Step 21. Alternative anastomotic site (2). Place a partially occluding, side-biting vascular clamp on the IVC. Make a venotomy using a #11 blade and a Potts scissors (Fig. 13-20).

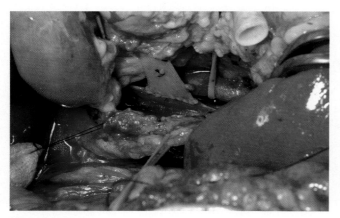

Figure 13-21.

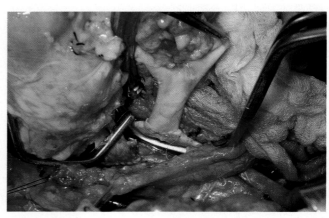

Figure 13-22.

Step 22. Alternative anastomotic site (3). Perform an end-to-side anastomosis of the graft portal vein to the IVC using 5-0 polypropylene suture (Fig. 13-21).

Step 23. Alternative anastomotic site (4). Clamp the mobilized common iliac artery in the recipient. Perform an end-to-side anastomosis between the stem of the Y-graft and the common iliac artery of the recipient. In Figure 13-22, the venous clamp has been moved up onto the portal vein off the IVC. If the pancreas is being transplanted in combination with a kidney transplant, many surgeons prefer to place the pancreas in the right iliac fossa and the kidney on the left. Alternatively, both grafts may be placed on the right. In this case, the pancreas graft is drained into the IVC with the Y-graft sewn end-to-side to the common iliac artery. The advantage of an all right-sided approach is speed; the self-retaining retractor does not need to be adjusted and the intestines do not need to be repacked.

Physiologic portal insulin delivery can be achieved by draining the graft portal vein into the recipient's SMV (technique not shown). Locate the SMV by lifting the transverse mesocolon superiorly and gently retracting the mesentery of the small bowel inferiorly. Palpate the pulse of the SMA. The SMV is lateral to the SMA (i.e., to the patient's right). Score the mesentery overlying the SMV. Using a right angle, ligate and divide the overlying tissue. The SMV is thin-walled, with fine branches that can be troublesome. They should be identified and suture-ligated with 6-0 polypropylene on the vessel. The operation then proceeds using a side-biting vascular clamp on the SMV for the end-to-side portal vein anastomosis. With SMV drainage, the Y-graft is tunneled through the ileal mesentery to the recipient common iliac artery. It may be necessary to add another segment of donor iliac vessel, such as a piece of external iliac artery that has been trimmed from the Y-graft, to achieve sufficient length. Although the superficial location of the SMV is technically appealing, the SMV may easily twist and pancreas graft positioning can be tricky, thereby courting the disaster of graft thrombosis.

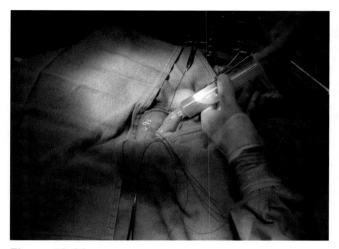

Figure 13-23.

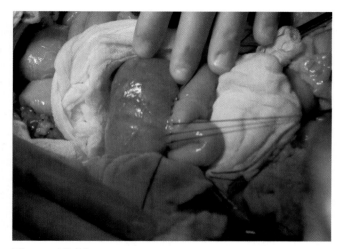

Figure 13-24.

Step 24. Donor duodenum decompression. While hemostasis is being established, remember that the duodenal segment is a closed loop and may rapidly fill with pancreatic secretions. To avoid a so-called Pfeffer loop (an experimental animal model in which a closed duodenal segment produces pancreatitis), aspirate the duodenal segment with a 16-gauge needle on a 50-cc piston syringe. Tunnel the needle under the serosa for 2 cm, then pass it through the mucosa into the lumen. This creates a valve that will minimize leakage upon withdrawal of the needle (Fig. 13-23).

Step 25. Enteric drainage of donor duodenum. To identify a loop of recipient bowel for enteric drainage of pancreatic secretions, identify the recipient's ligament of Treitz. Follow the small bowel distally until a loop of small bowel is found that rests side-to-side against the graft duodenum without tension. The more proximal small bowel is preferable because of its relative sterility. Too-distal drainage of exocrine secretions may cause diarrhea or exacerbate diabetic diarrhea. Clamp the recipient small bowel with bowel clamps until completion of the side-to-side duodeno-enteric (graft–recipient) anastomosis. Before opening the decompressed duodenum, pack the area around the graft off with wet laparotomy pads to catch any spillage. With the graft duodenum and the apex of the small bowel loop in contact, place a back row of 3-0 silk seromuscular sutures (Fig. 13-24).

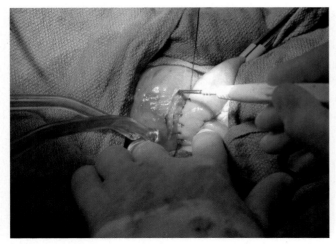

Figure 13-25.

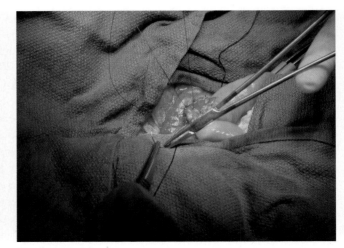

Figure 13-26.

Step 26. Enteric drainage of donor duodenum. Open the graft duodenum and apposing small bowel 4 to 6 cm using electrocautery. There are parallel full-thickness incisions through the bowel walls. Have suction ready to capture any bowel content from spilling and contaminating the general field (Fig. 13-25).

Step 27. Enteric drainage of donor duodenum (2). Complete the inner row of the back wall using full-thickness bites of 3-0 PDS. Convert the back wall over-and-over spiral stitch to a Connell stitch on the anterior wall (Fig. 13-26).

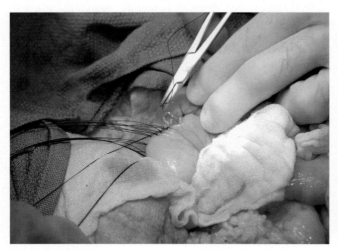

Figure 13-27.

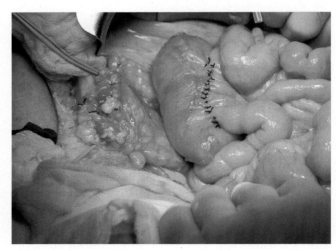

Figure 13-28.

Step 28. Enteric drainage of donor duodenum (3). Create a second outer layer of 3-0 silk seromuscular sutures. Remove the clamps (Fig. 13-27).

Step 29. Enteric drainage of donor duodenum (4). (Fig. 13-28). Alternatively, pass an end-to-end anastomosis (EEA) stapling device through the open distal end of the graft duodenum to create the duodeno-enteric anastomosis. There are other variations. A so-called omega loop (or uncut Roux loop) can be created with recipient small bowel by making a side-to-side entero-enterostomy, either stapled or hand-sewn. A TA staple line is placed transversely across the proximal recipient small bowel just beyond the anastomosis to defunctionalize the 16- to 20-cm loop. Other surgeons create a formal Roux-en-Y. In theory, an anastomosis to a defunctionalized omega or Roux limb would be less problematic should a leak occur.

Urinary bladder drainage of the pancreas (technique not shown) has lost favor. Patients often suffered from frequent dehydration and acidosis with this technique. In addition, urinary tract infections, hematuria, and urethritis in males were vexing problems. The purported advantage of urinary drainage—monitoring urinary amylase as a harbinger of rejection—has been supplanted in enterically drained grafts by percutaneous biopsy.

We do not routinely perform appendectomy in pancreas transplantation. Some advocate incidental appendectomy to avoid future confusion between appendicitis and graft pancreatitis or rejection.

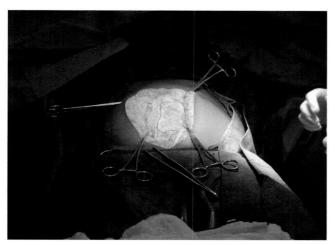

Figure 13-29.

Step 30. Abdominal closure. Before closing the abdomen, inspect the vascular anastomoses and the pancreas graft to ensure complete hemostasis. Close any mesenteric defects that represent potential sites for internal hernias. Evaluate the positioning of the pancreas, with particular attention to the portal vein, which should be straight and full. The splenic vein should be soft. A pulse is readily palpable in the tail of the pancreas. Then wash the peritoneal cavity with several liters of warm saline. Close the midline with running monofilament 1-0 PDS or polypropylene suture. Close the subcutaneous tissue and staple the skin. No drains are used. Dress the wound (Fig. 13-29).

Index